# YOUR EYES ARE YOUR WINDOW ON THE WORLD.
# KEEP THEM HEALTHY.

See better longer when you discover:

- ❑ How natural regeneration therapies can arrest and sometimes turn the degenerative process around

- ❑ What to look for in a pair of good-quality sunglasses—and why you should be wearing them

- ❑ How certain foods, substances, stress, and activities affect your body

- ❑ What kinds of foods and dietary supplements provide the greatest nutritional benefits for your eyes

- ❑ Ways to minimize the damaging effects of environmental toxins like cigarette smoke, sun, and pollutants

. . . and much more.

## SAVE YOUR SIGHT!

vitamin
Pg. 38
Pg. 53
& 54

# SAVE YOUR SIGHT!

## Natural Ways to Prevent and Reverse Macular Degeneration

Marc R. Rose, M.D.,
and Michael R. Rose, M.D.

WARNER BOOKS

A Time Warner Company

PUBLISHER'S NOTE: The information in this book can be a valuable addition to your doctor's advice, but it is not intended to replace the services of trained health professionals. You should consult your physician or health care professional in matters relating to your health, and in particular regarding symptoms that may require diagnosis or immediate attention.

Grateful acknowledgment is given to reprint "The Many Disguises of MSG" chart on pages 86–87: Reprinted with permission from *Excitotoxins: The Taste That Kills* by Russell L. Blaylock, M.D., Health Press, Santa Fe, NM, 1994.

Warner Books, Inc., 1271 Avenue of the Americas, New York, NY 10020

Visit our Web site at http://warnerbooks.com

A Time Warner Company

Printed in the United States of America

First Printing: August 1998

10 9 8 7 6 5 4 3 2 1

Library of Congress Cataloging-in-Publication Data

Rose, Marc R.
    Save your sight! : natural ways to prevent and reverse macular degeneration / Marc R. Rose and Michael R. Rose.
        p.   cm.
    Includes bibliographical references.
    ISBN 0-446-67402-8
    1. Retinal degeneration—Alternative treatment.  2. Eye—Diseases— Alternative treatment.  I. Rose, Michael R., M.D.  II. Title.
RE661.D3R67   1998
617.7—dc21                                            97-41030
                                                        CIP

*Book design by Nancy Singer Olaguera*
*Text composition by Peng Olaguera*
*Illustrations by Tu Pham*

---

**ATTENTION: SCHOOLS AND CORPORATIONS**

WARNER books are available at quantity discounts with bulk purchase for educational, business, or sales promotional use. For information, please write to: SPECIAL SALES DEPARTMENT, WARNER BOOKS, 1271 AVENUE OF THE AMERICAS, NEW YORK, NY 10020

*Dedicated to our children,*
*Adam, Joanna, Alyssa, Jonathan, Hillary,*
*David, Sara, Stephen, Jennifer, and Jerry,*
*who have inspired us*
*to search more deeply*
*for the answers.*

# Acknowledgments

We would like to thank Bill Sardi for his years of research into the intricacies of nutrition and eye diseases, and hence his invaluable contribution to this book. We would also like to thank Virginia Hopkins for her role in helping us envision, write, and edit this book, and Melissa Lowenstein for her expertise in tracking down the latest research and putting it all down on the written page. We owe much appreciation to our editor, Colleen Kapklein, who saw the value of this book and guided us to create a timely and clear work. We are indebted to the courageous and pioneering work of the late Linus Pauling, and to Jonathan Wright, M.D., and Alan Gaby, M.D., for their pioneering work in nutritional therapy in medical practice.

# Contents

# Introduction

## You Can Keep Your Vision Sharp as You Age

Macular degeneration is a devastating disease of progressive loss of vision and, for many, eventual blindness. In spite of the fact that it is the leading cause of blindness among older Americans, it has not attracted a lot of research money or media attention until recently. Some twelve million people show the early telltale signs of macular degeneration, and four million people already suffer from loss of vision.

Why don't we have an American Macular Degeneration Society, or a department at the National Institutes of Health devoted to a war on macular degeneration? Perhaps the reason is that those who are afflicted by macular degeneration are older, or that loss of vision tends to make people retreat into themselves, rather than stand up and shout for attention. Mainstream medicine has no effective drug or surgical treatment for it, so who wants to talk about that?

We are both ophthalmologists, medical doctors who specialize in the prevention and healing of diseases of the eyes. To help our patients save their sight, we have also become research scientists, working to understand how the health of the eyes and body are interconnected. Our quest to find answers for our patients suffering from a long list of eye diseases, including glaucoma, cataracts, diabetic eye disease, and retinitis pigmentosa, has led us into the world of alternative medicine. You'll be amazed at how relatively simple the answers are. There are no magic pills, no exotic new technologies (which we love, but they don't apply here) or fancy diets that will prevent and stop eye disease. The answers are found in sensible diet, nutritional supplements, exercise, and some important lifestyle choices. And best of all, there are no drug side effects or the risks associated with surgery.

We have seen hundreds of patients halt the progression of macular degeneration, and dozens actually reverse it. Most doctors don't yet embrace the kind of nutritional therapies described in this book; we hope that they come around soon.

Chances are good that you bought this book because you or someone close to you has been diagnosed with eye disease. If you are one of the millions with macular degeneration, your eye doctor most likely has told you there is nothing to be done short of risky laser surgery to slow your loss of vision. We know you are looking for another path to better eye health. We're glad you've found this book.

We're going to give you very detailed nutritional guidelines that we have seen prevent, halt, and sometimes even reverse the progress of macular degeneration and other eye diseases related to aging. If you can commit to our Ten Steps to Restoring Vision and Vitality and the nutritional protocol for your eye disease for at least nine months, you can almost certainly improve your vision. At the very least, you can keep it from getting worse.

Best of all, your vision isn't the only thing that will get better. The recommendations you'll find in this book will improve the health of your entire body. What's good for your eyes is good for all of you.

It's never too early or too late to take the steps we recommend. Eye disease and other diseases that afflict aging people begin in your twenties and thirties, and no matter how old you are, your health can always improve.

# 1

# Your Eyes Are a Window to Your Health: Ten Steps to Restoring Vision and Vitality

An eye exam reveals much more than the condition of your eyes. They are a window to the inner workings of your body, and a barometer of how healthy you are. When we look into the eye with a special instrument that allows a view beneath the surface, we can check the blood vessels behind the retina. If they are affected by disease, seen as tiny clots in the capillaries there, it's probable that blood vessels throughout the body are similarly afflicted. If the optic nerve is pale from lack of blood flow, we can make the same assumption. The effects of high blood cholesterol can be seen in the form of a grey ring around the inside of the clear cornea. If the iris is inflamed, it's a safe bet that there is inflammation elsewhere in the body.

There are many eye problems that reflect ill health in the body that can often be prevented or stopped in a matter of months with appropriate diet, supplements, and lifestyle changes. These include age spots on the retina known as *drusen* (an early sign of macular degeneration), ophthalmic migraines (squiggly flashes of light seen in the peripheral vision), Bitot's spots (on the whites of the eyes), poor night vision, floaters, chronic glare and light sensitivity, eye hemorrhages, cataracts, dry eyes, and macular edema (swelling).

In many cases, symptoms that crop up in the eyes are the first sign of diseases in other body parts. We often discover signs of diabetes, high blood pressure, blood vessel disease, or autoimmune disorders in the process of examining a patient's eyes.

If you have any of the symptoms of eye disease described in this book, please see your eye doctor immediately. The earlier you detect and diagnose eye disease, the easier it is to halt its progression and even reverse it. We recommend yearly eye exams, and if you have any progressive eye disease such as cataracts, macular degeneration, or glaucoma, we recommend checkups every six months.

## Ten Steps to Restoring Vision and Vitality

It follows that if you take the necessary steps to prevent eye disease or keep it from worsening, your whole body will enjoy the benefits. We've boiled the fundamentals of our approach down to Ten Steps to Restoring Vision and Vitality. These ten steps give you a foundation to build on. They provide guidelines that are tried, true, and supported by scientific research as well as our personal experiences with the people in our medical practice. Using the ten steps as a base, you can add our recommendations for specific eye problems found in the rest of the book, and summarized in Appendix I.

Most of the ten steps won't be new to you, but we hope they serve to give you a new attitude toward your health. We live by these guidelines, and although they can prove a challenge at first, the way you'll feel after a few months will make following them all worthwhile. No matter what the state of your health is now, we promise that if you follow these ten steps, your health will improve.

We want to emphasize, though, that we're putting the responsibility for your health into your hands. Modern medicine has made us feel as though we must hand over all control of our health to our doctors. We expect a magical elixir or surgery to fix what ails us. Our prescription gives you the tools—physically, emotionally, mentally, and even spiritually—for improving your health every moment of every day. You're going to enhance your body's innate ability to resist illness and aging. The best we can do is give you the tools; it's up to you to put them to use. It's well worth the effort, and your eyes will show you the difference.

Our ten secrets to restoring vision and vitality aren't necessarily in order of importance. Each one has equal weight, and you decide which to incorporate into your life first. Personally, we believe that if you adopt the first two steps, the rest will be much easier. The steps related to diet, nutrition, and exercise will be covered in detail in their own chapters.

### 1. Cultivate awareness; have a spiritual practice.

The first secret to great health is noticing what makes you healthy and what makes you sick. Cultivate awareness by becoming conscious of what you're doing and thinking. A good place to begin cultivating awareness is with your eating habits.

You're probably used to eating whatever is in front of you without much thought. Next time you're pulling into the drive-through for a burger, think for a moment. First, make certain you're actually hungry. Often we eat simply because it's lunchtime or dinnertime, or we have a craving, or we're bored or procrastinating. If you are indeed hungry, ask yourself whether a glass of cool, clear water and some fruit or a salad might be a better choice. Maybe it's not, maybe your body could use some protein and fat right now. The point is to be aware of what you're doing.

Next time you automatically plop onto the couch, remote in hand, ask yourself whether there's anything you really want to watch on TV. Would you feel better if you got up and went outdoors? Maybe you do need to vegetate in front of the TV for an hour or two, but consider a walk, a phone call with a loved one, or a good book.

We believe it's important to have a spiritual practice that gives you a sense of a higher meaning to life. When you have a sense of purpose, of mission, of meaning in your life, everything you do is enhanced by that point of view. All the better if your spiritual practice includes some form of meditation.

Meditation can be a wonderful way to bring yourself daily into a place of calm, peace, and balance, which is good for every cell in your body. In fact, even if it's not a part of your spiritual practice, we recommend you take up some type of meditative practice. It doesn't have to be sitting still and chanting an inward tone. It could be yoga, Tai Chi, or qi gong, all meditative practices combined with physical movement.

## 2. Everything in moderation.

These ten steps are not about eating only rice and vegetables, or meditating for hours on end, nor are they about ignoring your sugar and fat intake and giving in to the urge to be a couch potato. We're striving for something more balanced, which we call moderation.

It's not easy to live a health-conscious lifestyle in our culture. Friends and family may not understand or accept your new lifestyle. If you must skip a few days of exercise, eat a piece of sugary birthday cake, or sit in a smoky room with dear friends, don't let it throw you. Simply go back to doing things healthfully. Feeling guilty or angry is counterproductive.

On the other hand, there are those of you who think that if some lifestyle modification is good, more must be better. These ambitious souls are the ones who start their exercise program with a ten-mile run and resolve to ingest nothing but alfalfa sprouts and vitamin pills. That won't work, either, because it won't last.

What we're working for here is a long-term healthy lifestyle that is balanced. Ease into these changes. Find out what works best for you. Take one step at a time. Diets and lifestyle changes that are extremely unbalanced inevitably result in imbalance in your body.

The results of very-low-calorie diets for weight loss provide a good lesson on the wisdom of the body: It thinks you're in a famine, and slows your metabolism down to compensate. When you begin to eat normally again, your body needs fewer calories and stores the rest as fat. The dieter ends up gaining the weight back plus a couple of extra pounds!

Moderate exercise enhances immune function (see Chapter 12). Immoderate exercise depresses it. Intense, frequent exercise also greatly increases the rate at which your body produces unstable molecules called free radicals. (See Chapter 2 for more information on free radicals.) What constitutes "immoderation?" That will vary from person to person. Again, notice what makes you tired, what makes you energetic. Develop your own awareness of what moderation means to you.

### 3. Enjoy eating a variety of fresh, natural foods and cultivate good digestion.

Yes, you are what you eat, but you are also *how* you eat, so we want eating to be fun and enjoyable for you. Let's skip the yo-yo diets and strict, boring regimens, and find a balance that's both healthful and delicious.

When we eat too much food, it often is because we're not paying attention as we eat. We want you to enjoy every bite. As you eat your food, relish it. Enjoy the flavors, textures, and aromas. Give thanks for such a delicious meal. Take the time to have a leisurely meal. This is nourishment not only for your body but for your soul as well.

Eat a variety of foods so you'll get a variety of nutrients and add enjoyment to your meal. Experiment with different ethnic cuisines. Make your plate colorful. Eat red, orange, yellow, and green vegetables. Try steaming, stir frying, baking, and grilling vegetables.

When we recommend "natural" foods, we mean as close as possible to the way they were designed by Mother Nature:

- Whole grains
- Fresh pesticide-free organic fruits and vegetables

- Meat and dairy products untainted by antibiotics and hormones
- Fresh fish baked, poached, grilled, or broiled (not fried).

If you eat fresh, natural foods, chances are your digestion will be good, but as we age, our ability to secrete digestive enzymes and absorb nutrients diminishes. Later, in Chapter 9, we'll give you a list of supplements to take if your digestion could use some help.

## 4. Drink plenty of clean water throughout the day, every day.

This is pretty easy so far, isn't it? And how wonderful that something as simple as drinking clean water every day can keep you looking and feeling young and vibrant. We recommend at least six to eight glasses of water a day (eight-ounce glasses).

If you have any doubt whatsoever that drinking plenty of clean water is one of the healthiest steps you can take, please read the book *Your Body's Many Cries for Water*, by F. Batmanghelidj, M.D. He makes a convincing case that we are chronically dehydrated, and that many of our degenerative diseases can be cured simply by drinking more water.

We do recommend that you invest in a water filter. In the past decade America has developed polluted tap water along with the rest of the world. You need to filter aluminum, heavy metals such as lead, benzenes from petrochemical pollution, chlorine, fluoride, and parasites such as *Giardia* and cryptosporidium, which aren't killed by water plant treatment. (You will need a special filter to get rid of fluoride, but if you have arthritis, heart disease, or osteoporosis, it may be worth it. Fluoride is nearly everywhere in our food and water, so what we get in the water supply becomes excessive, contributing to the above chronic diseases. Adults do not need fluoride! We recommend that at the very least you use a non-fluoride toothpaste.)

When you drink plenty of water you'll notice that your skin is clearer, you'll be more "regular," and you'll have less appetite for junk food. If you tend to retain water, drinking more may be just what the doctor ordered. Your body, when dehydrated, will retain water so that it can survive what it perceives to be a drought.

The thirst mechanism isn't always a reliable measure of when or how much you need to drink, especially in older people. Make drinking plenty of water a habit and stick to it. And by the way, only water counts as water. Soda, juice, coffee, and tea don't count, nor do alcoholic beverages.

5. **Take nutritional supplements every day, and, as you age, take advantage of natural regeneration therapies.**

Most of you probably take a daily multivitamin that you buy at the supermarket or drugstore.

The typical drugstore brands contain only the Recommended Dietary Allowance (RDA) of the vitamins and minerals. These allowances are for the minimum daily intake required for the prevention of deficiency diseases such as scurvy, pellagra, and rickets. We're guiding you to clarity, longevity, youthfulness, and better vision, so we want you to do *way* better than the RDA.

The environment you live in is constantly pulling on your body's vitamin resources. For example, stress, air pollution, pesticides, alcohol, and bad food will deplete vitamins. Taking supplements is your way of counteracting the emotional and physical stressors of everyday life.

You can also self-treat a tremendous variety of ailments safely and effectively with supplements. If you feel yourself coming down with a cold or flu, you can take vitamin C, echinacea, and zinc, and avoid getting sick altogether or shorten the duration and severity of the symptoms. If your joints are aching, you can take glucosamine sulfate. If you're having muscle spasms at night, you can take a calcium/magnesium supplement before you go to bed. These remedies are safe, gentle, and effective *and* treat the underlying cause, not the symptom. This is the future of medicine. Jump on the bandwagon now, and you'll be healthier and happier for it.

The goal of using natural regeneration therapies is to supplement what is declining in an aging body. Therapies include naturally occurring versions of your body's own hormones, as well as supplements with proven anti-aging and lifespan-extending effects. These therapies go beyond simple maintenance of good health and can add energetic years to your life. This is where the miracles of science work to augment the miracles of the body.

The hormones we recommend for our patients include DHEA (dehydroepiandrosterone), pregnenolone, progesterone, estrogens, testosterone, melatonin, and human growth hormone. Some of the anti-aging supplements are ubiquinone (also known as coenzyme Q10), ginseng, chromium, selenium, betaine hydrochloride, vitamin E, vitamin A, and magnesium. Although we won't be covering these hormones and supplements in this book in detail, we recommend you take advantage of the "Recommended Reading" list in Appendix II to find out more.

## 6. Make exercise part of your daily renewal.

You don't want to go to the gym or take a yoga class? Take a walk. It doesn't get much simpler than this, does it?

The human body is beautifully designed for movement. If you deprive it of exercise, it gets stiff and painful. Cholesterol levels, blood pressure, joint health, and emotional health are negatively impacted. As soon as you adopt a mild to moderate exercise program, you'll notice improved mood and better sleep. It doesn't take a high-intensity, no-pain-no-gain program; in fact, you'll be a lot more likely to quit completely if exercise is unpleasant.

If you can't walk for an hour, try a half-hour. If a half-hour isn't manageable, take fifteen minutes. Something is always better than nothing when it comes to exercise. If you can walk for five minutes six times a day, you're doing enough to gain significant health benefits.

7. **Minimize your exposure to toxins, poisons, and pollutants.**

Any substance that can do damage to your body, and in doing so contributes to the development of pain and illness, fits our definition of toxin, poison, or pollutant.

We humans have made the sad and tragic mistake of fouling our nest and creating pervasive pollution on the earth. It's nearly inescapable. The best you can do, short of holing up on an unspoiled desert island or adding a gas mask and latex gloves to your beauty regimen, is to eliminate the major sources of toxins from your life.

- Don't smoke.
- Don't hang around with people who are smoking.
- Don't exercise on heavily trafficked city streets.
- Do buy organic foods.
- Do install a water filter in your kitchen faucet.

- Don't use pesticides, herbicides, or fungicides (throw away your cans of insect spray and weed killer).
- Don't eat highly processed foods. (Here's a good rule: If you don't recognize or can't pronounce an ingredient on the label, leave it on the shelf.)
- Do avoid over-the-counter and prescription drugs as possible. (See step 8 for details.)
- Do buy carpets and furniture that are free of fumes.

## 8. Beware of drugs.

Our problems with street drugs in America are nothing compared to our problems with prescription drugs. At least 140,000 people die in hospitals each year from misprescribed prescription drugs, and many hundreds of thousands more are hospitalized. This costs us billions of dollars in health care and causes incalculable damage to people's lives, and yet it's all perfectly legal.

Nobody is more aware than we doctors are that prescription drugs can be lifesavers in some instances. Antibiotics have saved many lives. Painkillers allow suffering people to rest in comfort. But, these days, our guess is that drugs are killing as many people as they're helping, and they are dramatically reducing the quality of life for millions of others. We assure you they are doing very little to improve your health that can't be done with less money, fewer side effects, and vastly better results using more down-to-earth remedies.

Unfortunately, the typical doctor practicing today is under enormous time and energy constraints. He or she has to see more patients than ever before to keep a practice afloat, so it's much more time-efficient to get a list of symptoms and scribble out a prescription than to address the whole person and the possible root of the illness.

The bottom line is that your doctor is a human being, not a deity. That prescription he or she's handing you really may not be necessary. Always ask for a nondrug alternative, and do your own homework.

Best of all, find a physician or a health care professional such as a chiropractor or naturopathic doctor who will work with you to prevent illness and maintain your health.

**9. Wear good sunglasses whenever you're out in the midday sun for more than ten to fifteen minutes.**

You'll discover as you read this book that overexposure to the sun, combined with too few antioxidants and too many toxins, is likely the leading underlying cause of many of our age-related eye diseases. Conscientiously wearing sunglasses that protect your eyes from ultraviolet light can add years of clear vision to your life. You'll read about sunglasses in detail in Chapter 14.

Apply the principle of moderation here too, and don't go to extremes with the sunglasses. While too much sun is destructive, too little isn't good, either. Sunlight is a nutrient, and your eyes need it just as much as the rest of your body does. Let your eyes have some exposure to the sun every day, preferably in the morning or late afternoon, and wear your sunglasses the rest of the time.

## 10. Cultivate fun, balanced healthy relationships with people you love.

How are your relationships with the people in your life? Are there people you can talk with freely about your thoughts and feelings? Do you have a spouse, a relative, a friend, or even a pet to love and care for?

Humans by their nature are social and need healthy relationships with others in order to thrive. People who have pets, who volunteer for good causes, and who are in stable, happy marriages live longer and healthier lives than people who are withdrawn, lonely, and depressed. We even have studies showing that volunteering to help others is good for the heart.

Sometimes it can take a huge effort to get up off the couch or out of bed and "do," but doing for others is one of the best cures we know for whatever ails you.

## IN SHORT . . . TEN STEPS TO RESTORING VISION AND VITALITY

1. Cultivate awareness; have a spiritual practice.
2. Everything in moderation.
3. Enjoy eating a variety of fresh, natural foods and cultivate good digestion.
4. Drink plenty of clean water through the day, every day.
5. Take nutritional supplements every day, and, as you age, take advantage of natural regeneration therapies.
6. Make exercise part of your daily renewal.
7. Minimize your exposure to toxins, poisons, and pollutants.
8. Beware of drugs.
9. Wear good sunglasses whenever you're out in the midday sun for more than ten to fifteen minutes.
10. Cultivate fun, balanced, healthy relationships with people you love.

# 2

# How Your Eyes Work

The more you understand about how your eyes work and what can go wrong, the better you'll understand the importance of the nutritional and lifestyle "pre-scriptions" we're giving you. But before we take a look at the eyes themselves, let's get better acquainted with an important biological process that can make all the difference between sharp and fuzzy vision.

An imbalance between free radicals created by oxidation reactions and the antioxidants that neu-tralize them is one of the common threads of cause and effect that is woven through all of the major eye diseases and nearly all of the disabilities and diseases we associate with aging. Some researchers go so far as to connect all disease processes directly or indi-rectly with oxidation.

## Quenching the Fires of Oxidation

Oxidation reactions occur when oxygen reacts with something in the body or the environment that creates unstable molecules called free radicals. Free radicals bounce around looking for something to latch on to, but unless they latch on to an antioxidant, they'll make whatever they latch on to unstable in turn, creating a chain reaction.

For example, a free radical that encounters an unsaturated fat will latch on to it and oxidize it, turning it rancid. A free radical in an apple with a bite out of it will start an oxidation reaction that turns the apple's flesh brown. If you sprinkle lemon juice, which contains the antioxidant vitamin C, on the apple, it won't turn brown because the vitamin C will neutralize the free radicals and stop the oxidation process. Free radicals cause many types of cell damage, even to the point of damaging DNA, the cells' genetic coding system.

One of your primary sources of free radicals is your own body. For example, your body is always burning fuel (from food) with the aid of oxygen molecules that are brought to all cells by way of the blood vessels. When the oxygen is used, comparable to the burning of fuel in a car, what's left is a mixture that includes free radicals. Oxidation reactions are happening millions of times a second in your body, but you have a sophisticated array of antioxidants that, in a healthy body, are on the spot to neutralize any excess free radicals.

The free radicals in your body play some positive roles too. They have important roles as messengers between cells and in enzyme reactions, and the immune system uses them to kill unwanted invaders.

Your body can make some of these antioxidants

(glutathione, melatonin, and coenzyme Q10 are examples), while others are part of the foods you eat (vitamins A, C, E, and selenium are a few of these). Once the antioxidant balances the free radical, it either remains neutral or is reactivated by another antioxidant. The antioxidants all work synergistically, each enhancing and supporting the effects of the other.

Free radical formation is accelerated by radiation, cigarette smoke, car exhaust, and a wide variety of other environmental toxins such as pesticides, herbicides, and solvents. When we take these substances into our bodies, the extra free radical load can overwhelm our antioxidant defenses.

Disease and aging begin when there are more free radicals than antioxidants. In an environment filled with toxins, this happens fairly easily. Western lifestyles, with high levels of stress, poor diets of processed foods, and little attention paid to the needs of the body (until something goes wrong), predispose us to this oxidation imbalance. If your diet doesn't contain all the elements needed to defend against free radical assault, your body will suffer.

## Inflammation and Your Eyes

If you aren't getting the right nutrients, eye diseases can result. One of the links between poor nutrition and disease is the inflammatory response.

Inflammation is a natural process your body uses to heal damaged cells, and it's intricately connected with the process of free radical damage (oxidation).

Sometimes, if there are nutritional deficiencies or toxins in the picture, the inflammatory response can get out of control and fluid pressure around the inflammation rises above what it should be. High fluid pressure and other aspects of an out-of-control inflammatory response are harmful to the body's tissues. A lifetime of poor nutrition and exposure to toxins tips the delicately balanced inflammatory response from health-preserving to health-threatening.

Think of the allergic response: When hay fever sufferers come into contact with something seemingly as harmless as fresh-cut flowers, they are thrown into sneezing fits, with runny nose and eyes, hives, or perhaps even lung congestion or constriction. That response is inflammatory and is controlled by a very complex system of checks and balances within the systems of the body.

Another example is arthritis: The joints become chronically inflamed, and connective tissue is destroyed as a result. Our nutritional prescriptions will help keep inflammation at bay.

## Caring for the Eyes Means Caring for the Rest of You

The good news is that if problems like macular degeneration, cardiovascular disease, cancer, arthritis, and stroke are at least in part caused by free-radical damage and inflammation, it follows that conscientious work towards self-protection against excessive oxidation means self-protection on all fronts. That's very different from the usual medical approach, where a drug given to cure one illness is likely to bring on another one, for which another drug is given, and so on and on and on. Keep this in mind as you read along.

## Just a Little Bit of Eye Anatomy

Light rays coming into the eye first pass through the cornea, a dense and curved clear layer. They move in from the cornea through a thick fluid (the *aqueous humor*) to the eye lens, which is right behind the iris and looks to us like the black circle of the pupil. The

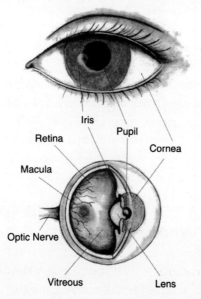

A frontal and three-quarter view of the human eye and the optic nerve, macula, retina, iris, pupil, cornea, lens, and vitreous.

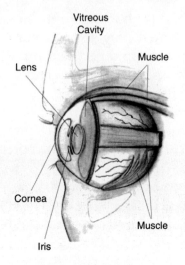

A side view of the human eye.

light continues to travel through the body of the eye, which is filled with more thick fluid (the *vitreous humor*). It then strikes the retina, which contains color-vision cells (rods and cones), spatial vision cells (at the fovea), protective pigment such as melanin, and cells that translate light into nerve impulses to be sent to the brain by way of the optic nerve.

## Ultraviolet and Blue Light: What's Harmful, What's Helpful

Light is a nutrient. Without light stimulation, the retina would shrink and become inactive. The same aphorism applies to the eyes as to the muscles, "Use it or lose it."

Not only is light what allows us to see the world around us, but it plays other roles in keeping the body in balance. It stimulates the production of certain hormones in the pituitary gland, which activate the adrenal glands on top of the kidneys. Cataracts that are severe enough to block most light from hitting the retina actually cause ankle and foot swelling because the hormonal messengers responsible for maintaining fluid balance in the body don't get their orders, expressed in the form of light.

The absence of light stimulates the secretion of the hormone melatonin, which sends the signal to the body that it's time to sleep. All sorts of regenerative processes happen while you sleep, and it's important that the quality of that sleep is good. Without the light of day, the internal clock gets thrown off. Melatonin may not be secreted at the right time, and sleep will be poor; this will affect how you feel when you're awake.

Vitamin D is manufactured in the body when it's exposed to ultraviolet light. Without vitamin D, calcium metabolism is impaired and bone health suffers. A few minutes of skin exposure to unfiltered sunlight can produce enough vitamin D to last for days or weeks, stored in the liver.

Ultraviolet (UV) light also can do harm, especially to the eyes. Studies show that UV rays promote cataracts, eyelid skin cancer, snow and sun blindness, abnormal growths on the surface of the eyes called *pterygia*, macular degeneration, and a form of melanoma that affects the back of the eyes. Since ultraviolet radiation from the sun is a major source of damage to the eyes from oxidation, we'd like you to protect your eyes from the sun, especially as you age.

No matter what the health of your eyes, we recommend that you invest in a pair of sunglasses that blocks out 100 percent of the UV-A and UV-B sun rays and that filters out at least 85 percent of blue-violet sun rays, and wear them whenever you'll be out in the sun for more than about fifteen minutes in the middle of the day. If you're squinting after your eyes have had time to adjust to the sunlight for a while, put on your sunglasses.

Many of the sunglasses sold are mislabeled. Talk with your eye doctor; he or she may be able to suggest a good local vendor to you. A hat with a brim is also good insurance for the health of your eyes.

Blue light is part of the visible spectrum. Too much blue light can harm your eyes by dramatically increasing the rate of formation of free radicals. Overexposure to blue light causes harmful deposits in the network of blood vessels feeding the retina. To be protected from retinal damage, choose lenses that filter at least some blue light. When you wear them the sky should appear somewhat grey.

Sunlight is like everything else in life, best enjoyed in moderation. Because sunlight also nourishes the eyes, I wouldn't suggest you wear sunglasses at all times unless you have advanced eye disease, but be smart. Enjoy the sunshine but don't overdo it, and remember to wear your sunglasses when it's bright. (See also Chapter 14, "Basic Eye Care," for more information on sunglasses.)

# 3

# The Nutritional Care and Feeding of Your Eyes

So far you've heard a lot about the powerful negative or positive effects your diet can have on the health of your eyes. Of our Ten Steps to Restoring Vision and Vitality, four of them relate to making foods, fluids, and nutritional supplements part of your daily renewal. Now we're going to give you very detailed guidelines on nutrients that can help you maintain good eyesight and information on why they work the way they do.

An eye-healthy diet begins with a diet that's rich in vitamins, minerals, complex carbohydrates, essential proteins and fats, as well as plenty of clean water. We're not going to recommend you eat a diet extremely low in fat or extremely high in protein or carbohydrates. These extremes might work for the one person in one hundred with a specific condition, but for the rest of us, balance is key. You can't eliminate all the fat in your diet without sacrificing essential nutrients. Too much protein can damage your kidneys. Too many carbohydrates will pack on the pounds.

Since carbohydrates have been the subject of much controversy lately, let's take a closer look at them.

## Not All Carbohydrates Are Created Equal

Look in your cupboards and try to identify all the carbohydrates. You might be surprised at the wide variety of foods that fall into this category. The box of sugared cereal, the can of peas, the bag of potatoes, the canister of brown sugar, the box of pasta, the loaf of French bread, the fat-free chips and crackers, the bag of apples and the jar of raw honey all contain carbohydrates. These foods are broken down into glucose, the simplest form of sugar.

Carbohydrates are an efficient fuel source because they are converted easily to glucose and thus to energy, but if you eat more carbohydrates than you burn off, they will stick with you as fat. That's right. Sugar, potatoes, and bread all are converted to fat if you don't use them fairly quickly for fuel. Fat will make you fat, and so will carbohydrates. But not all carbohydrates are created equal.

There is an important difference between the peas, potatoes, and apples on the one hand, and the honey, cereal, brown sugar, chips, crackers, pasta, and white bread on the other. The first group consists of *un*refined carbohydrates, close to the form in which nature made them, while the second group consists of refined carbohydrates created by heating, stripping, and milling of whole foods. Refined and processed foods are stripped of their vitamins, minerals, enzymes, and fiber. Preservatives, food dyes, and flavoring agents such as monosodium glutamate (MSG), sugar, and salt are added back in.

A white-flour bagel will provide you with energy from glucose, but it will give you next to nothing in the way of vitamins, minerals, essential oils, or fiber. When you eat that bagel, your body has to pull from stored nutrients to supply the materials needed to digest and metabolize it. If it had been a bagel made from fresh whole grains, seeds, and nuts, those nutrients would be part of the food itself. Processed foods and sugar have been called "anti-nutrients" because they actually drain nutrients instead of contributing them.

At the other end of the spectrum, the carbohydrates found in whole grains, fruits, vegetables, and legumes (beans) are broken down to glucose slowly and supply needed nutrients on the way. Their fiber slows digestion and provides a steady supply of glucose.

Refined sugars and flours are, in effect, predigested and quickly flood the bloodstream with glucose. Your pancreas releases the hormone insulin to carry the glucose out of the blood and into the cells, but in response to the spike of glucose the pancreas senses a crisis. It releases so much insulin that your blood is cleared of all its glucose and your blood glucose level dives, leaving you feeling exhausted and craving more sugar and refined carbohydrates to kick it back up again.

Day after day, week after week, year after year—a history of these fluctuations takes its toll. Dropping blood sugar brings on a  sharp increase in adrenal "fight or flight" hormones. These hormones work to mobilize stored fat and carbohydrates to keep you going until your next meal. It's a response designed to supply you with the energy to gather some more edible plants or hunt down an antelope. When refined carbohydrates are in the picture, blood sugar dips precipitously several times a day and the adrenals have to work hard to compensate. There's some evidence that this can result in exhaustion of the adrenal glands as well as of the parts of the pancreas that make insulin.

Carbohydrates have been touted for years as the answer to good nutrition and weight loss, yet Americans have grown fatter and fatter. This is because carbohydrates have calories, too! Yes, even complex carbohydrates have calories, and if you eat more than you burn off, you'll put on weight. The lesson of course is moderation. Make complex carbohydrates a balanced part of your meals and snacks so you can deliver nutrients with your calories.

## Not All Fats Are Created Equal

Conventional wisdom has urged you for years to replace saturated fats (solid at room temperature) like butter, lard, and coconut oil with polyunsaturated fats (liquid at room temperature) such as safflower and corn oil. But this so-called wisdom is more related to the politics of the processed food industry than to reality; polyunsaturated fats can be just as harmful to your health as the saturated fats.

Polyunsaturated oils are highly unstable and thus are extremely susceptible to oxidation. You know this as rancid oil. Chances are, that clear new bottle of vegetable oil is already rancid as you open it, and it's guaranteed to be within days of being opened. These highly oxidized oils run amuck in the body, oxidizing virtually everything they touch and putting a great burden on your antioxidant supply to stop the chain reaction. Rancid oils directly contribute to the clogging of small blood vessels, including those in the eye.

The essential fatty acids found in unprocessed vegetable oils are very necessary to good health but you need them only in very small amounts. The ideal way to get these oils is by eating plenty of fresh vegetables, fruits, nuts, and whole grains, where they are naturally preserved and stabilized by antioxidants such as vitamins A, E, and C.

Saturated fats are very stable. They don't oxidize easily. In light of the new evidence that oxidized oils shoulder some of the blame for the blood vessel injuries that lead to heart disease, we advise you to choose small amounts of saturated fats over polyunsaturates. If you eat saturated fats in excess, you will also get yourself in trouble. As always, moderation is your guide to good health.

The best of both worlds is found in monounsaturated oils such as those derived from olives, rape-seeds (the source of canola oil), and avocados. These are stable and contain essential oils your body needs to function properly. Olive oil has shown promise as a heart disease fighter. As you'll discover in Chapter 10, anything that promotes blood vessel health helps not only your heart but your eyes as well.

Cold-water fish like salmon, eaten twice weekly, safely supply unsaturated essential omega-3 oils. Studies showing the value of these oils in improving levels of "good" high-density lipoprotein (HDL) cholesterol, decreasing inflammation, and keeping artery disease at bay have been published in many medical journals.

The oils I want you to avoid as much as possible are the hydrogenated oils, also called trans fatty acids, found in margarine, chips, cookies, and most processed foods and baked goods. Trans fatty acids, identified on food labels as "partially hydrogenated," are partially saturated to address the problem of rancidity, but in the process of making them manufacturers have created a hybrid monster. These man-made oils have been linked directly to heart disease. They will do you no good and will not contribute to your nutrition. In fact I would classify them as anti-nutrients and even as toxins.

## The Cholesterol Controversy

For a couple of decades, mainstream medicine has been using multiple strategies to lower total blood cholesterol. Diets that restrict cholesterol-containing foods such as meats, eggs, and dairy products, plus barrages of cholesterol-lowering drugs, have been prescribed for millions of people, especially the elderly. Now it turns out that this approach has been misguided.

The reality is that the level of "bad" low-density lipoprotein (LDL) cholesterol in the blood hasn't been consistently linked to risk of heart disease, and your total blood cholesterol count is almost meaningless. What *is* important is that you have a healthy ratio of "good" HDL cholesterol to LDL cholesterol and that your LDL cholesterol not be oxidized. Drugs administered to lower cholesterol at all costs generally do more harm than good and have never been shown to reduce the risk of dying.

A high level of LDL cholesterol is a symptom of blood vessel disease rather than a cause of it. Cholesterol has gotten a bad rap, but it is a vital substance necessary for the transport of antioxidant substances to the eyes and other organs. It is the substance from which all of the steroid hormones are made, including testosterone, estrogen, progesterone, and DHEA. If you lower your cholesterol levels with drugs, without addressing the underlying problems causing the high levels in the first place, you'll suppress the symptoms, but your disease will continue to progress.

LDL cholesterol is not bad in and of itself. It is *oxidized* LDL cholesterol particles (also called *lipid peroxides*) that can clog your arteries and kill you. Although researchers haven't been able to directly

implicate the causes of LDL oxidation, the most educated guesses are that stress, low antioxidant levels,
and poor nutrition combined with exposure to toxins
such as pollution combine to throw LDL cholesterol
out of balance.

Rather than trying so hard to lower LDL cholesterol, it's much more important that you raise the
amount of "good" HDL naturally with exercise, plenty of garlic, soy protein, and omega-3 fatty acids
(found in deep-water fish). A glass or two of wine a
few times a week may help protect you from blood
vessel disease by raising your levels of HDL cholesterol. It's important, though, that you indulge with
moderation. A habit of more than two drinks of wine
daily leads to a large free-radical load, overwhelming
your antioxidant defenses.

If you suffer from eye disease, it's even more
important to be moderate with alcohol. Your liver
needs to be in tip-top shape to supply you with glutathione and vitamin A, both crucial for good eye
health.

## If You're Going to Have a Treat, Have a Healthy One

I don't know too many people who don't enjoy a
sweet treat now and then. But there are healthy
sweet treats and unhealthy sweet treats. If you're
going to treat yourself to ice cream, find a brand
that's made with whole ingredients, without all the
gums, emulsifiers, stabilizers, and colorings. All you

need to make ice cream is milk or cream, a little bit of sugar, and flavoring like fruit or chocolate. Do you prefer a chocolate bar to an ice cream cone? Find one made with cocoa butter and whole milk instead of hydrogenated oil and milk solids. Become a gourmet sweet eater and make it an occasional treat.

## Cultivate Healthy Eating Habits

One of the best moves you can make towards healthier eyes is to begin eating fresh, organic vegetables and fruits. Most communities these days have a local farmer's market in the summer and fall, stocked with colorful piles of organic, fresh-from-the-field produce. If you've been eating canned, frozen, and otherwise processed fruits and vegetables, eating fresh organic fruits and vegetables will be an incredible new taste sensation for you.

Produce that's not organic may look pretty because it's coated in wax, but it may be days or weeks old and low in vitamins. It may be contaminated with pesticides and grown in depleted soil that is low in essential minerals. Support your local farmer's market and tell your supermarket manager you want organic produce. It may cost a little more, but you're worth it!

Buy organic or hormone-free and drug-free meat, fish, and dairy products if at all possible. Otherwise they may be tainted by hormones and antibiotics that become concentrated in the fatty tissues of the animals that provide them.

Eat whole grains such as corn, rice, oats, millet, and barley, as well as legumes such as lentils, black beans, and soy products.

If you follow these guidelines, your diet will consist of foods in the form that nature intended. Cooking with these foods is easy because they taste so wonderful. With a few spices, vinegars, and healthy oils such as olive or canola, meals can be delicious, hearty, and nutritious.

Although there is a lot of conflicting information about the best way to eat, there are a few things we know for sure. We know that too much fat and sugar will make you sick and shorten your life and that eating lots of fresh vegetables will make you healthy and lengthen your life.

Our advice is to stay away from anything in a box, jar, or can whenever it's possible to do so. Studies that compare diseases show that people in countries like China, Japan, and India, whose diets are composed primarily of whole, unprocessed vegetable foods, suffer significantly less heart disease, arthritis, osteoporosis, and cancers of the breast, lung, and colon. When these people adopt a Western diet with lots of fat, processed foods, and sugar, they begin to develop the same diseases Americans do.

## Nutritional Supplements for the Health of Your Eyes

Many patients initially react the same way when we suggest they try nutritional supplements: "Oh, that's

okay, Dr. Rose, I eat a very good diet. I get all the vitamins I need." They often go on to say that they tried
a multivitamin for a while and didn't notice any difference in how they felt. Their other doctors have
told them that all a multivitamin could give them
was expensive urine. So they stopped taking them,
thinking it to be a waste of money. These people
aren't aware that most vitamin brands carried in
drugstores and supermarkets contain only a fraction
of the vitamins needed for optimal good health.

Linus Pauling, a biochemist who won two Nobel
prizes in his lifetime, would certainly have contested
the "I don't need vitamins" attitude. His ground-
breaking research on optimal vitamin supplementation for the prevention and treatment of disease was
the beginning of a nutritional revolution. In the early
1970s, when he began to look at studies about the
antiviral effects of vitamin C, he reasoned that people getting only the U.S. recommended dietary
allowance (RDA) were failing to tap the amazing
powers of megavitamin supplementation. Large
doses of vitamin C had already been shown to provide protection against the common cold. As Pauling
dug deeper, he learned that vitamin C, in doses
amounting to many times the RDA, could have positive effects on heart disease, eye diseases, cancer,
arthritis, and allergies, among other things. He
coined the term *orthomolecular medicine* to describe
the practice of preventing and treating disease with
"substances that are normally present in the body
and are required for good health."

The medical establishment is taking notice more

than twenty years later. Medical journals are dotted with studies about the ways in which natural substances might be used to combat aging and disease. Popular magazines and books are extolling the virtues of nutrient supplementation. Getting only the RDA of vitamins may protect you from diseases like scurvy (a vitamin C deficiency) or pellagra (a B vitamin deficiency), but you'll be missing out on the many other benefits of nutrient supplementation.

There's an exciting movement in today's science of nutrition from simply surviving to feeling great every day. Unfortunately, the medical establishment changes very slowly. Your doctor is still more likely to give you drugs than diet advice.

Even if you are enjoying good health at the moment, we recommend that you supplement the fresh, natural foods you eat with vitamins, especially if you are over the age of fifty, when your body needs extra nutritional support. We want you to be able to buffer all the toxins in the environment and have plenty of zip and zest left over to enjoy your life to the absolute fullest.

## Common Eye Problems That May Be Caused by Nutritional Deficiencies

Seemingly minor health problems in the body can be an indicator of bigger problems. For example, leg cramps and other muscle spasms can be an indication of magnesium deficiency, which in the long run can contribute directly to the development of heart disease. Digestive problems such as heartburn and gas can be an indicator of poor nutrient absorption. In the same way, common minor problems in the eyes can be an early indicator of nutritional deficiencies.

## Dry Eyes

Dry eyes, which are covered in more detail in Chapter 14, "Basic Eye Care," can be an indication of dehydration; or an allergy to pollens, foods, or cosmetics; or a deficiency of the fatty acid GLA (gamma-linolenic acid). If you also have dry hair, skin, and nails, you may need GLA oils. The usual culprit is overconsumption of hydrogenated oils, which block utilization of the essential fatty acids found in small amounts of fresh vegetables, nuts and seeds, and fish.

If you have dry eyes, you can try taking a supplement of borage oil, black currant seed oil, or evening primrose oil, all concentrated sources of GLA oils, for three months, while you cut back substantially on hydrogenated oils and increase your intake of fresh vegetables, nuts, and seeds.

## Floaters

If you ask most eye doctors about floaters, those annoying black or grey specks that drift across your vision, you'll be told they're harmless and not to worry. But in truth these clumps of cells floating in the vitreous jelly of your eye may be an indication that the collagen in your eye isn't as strong as it could be. The solution is to increase your intake of vitamin C, bioflavonoids, glucosamine sulfate, and copper, all of which play an important role in maintaining collagen strength. You can take an extra dose of 1,000 to 2,000 mg of vitamin C daily, 1,000 to 1,500 mg of glucosamine sulfate, and 200 to 400 mg of anthocyanidin bioflavonoids (such as bilberry or grapeseed), and be sure you're getting at least 5 mg of copper every day in your multivitamin or in a separate supplement.

## Bloodshot Eyes

We all have times when our eyes are bloodshot from too much sun, too little sleep, or exposure to dust, wind, pollen, or other allergens. But if your eyes are chronically bloodshot and you have ruled out the above causes, it may be that the delicate capillaries in your eyes are trying to tell you something. They're weak and allowing blood to leak out. For most people some extra vitamin C (1,000–2,000 mg daily) and bioflavonoids (200–400 mg daily) will help within a few weeks.

Other factors that can cause chronic bloodshot eyes are excessive estrogen, antihistamines, steroids, and chronic stress.

But be sure to read Chapter 10 on circulation and do everything you can to strengthen your circulatory system. Damaged and weak capillaries in your eyes are an early warning system that all is not well with your circulation.

## Poor Night Vision

Sometimes the inability to adjust to sudden darkness or bright light is an early warning sign that you have retinitis pigmentosa or macular degeneration; check with your eye doctor. If not such a condition, it could be a nutritional deficiency.

Your mother was right when she told you that if you ate your carrots, you could see better at night. The same goes for all orange, yellow, and deep green vegetables, which contain carotenoids that supply the eyes with vitamin A and other eye-nourishing nutrients. Poor night vision may be a symptom of a deficiency in omega-3 fatty acids, which can be cured by eating plenty of fish or taking fish oil supplements (well preserved with antioxidants, please!). If it takes your eyes a long time to adjust when you walk into a movie theater or out into bright sunlight from a darkened room, you can try taking some cod liver oil, which contains both omega-3 fatty acids and vitamin A, for a few months.

## Eyelid Twitch

An eyelid twitch is usually a muscle spasm and often can be treated effectively with magnesium. You can add 50 mg of vitamin $B_6$ daily until it goes away.

## Presbyopia: Do You Need Reading Glasses?

Somewhere between the ages of forty and fifty most of us start holding reading material at arm's length so it will come into focus, and we find we need more light to see small print; eventually we get reading glasses or bifocals. The condition responsible for these measures is known as *presbyopia*, and we think it happens because as we age the muscles around the lens of the eye, which is where we focus, become stretched out and less flexible, and the lens itself becomes less flexible and clear.

A good multivitamin and plenty of antioxidant vitamins are your cornerstones for postponing presbyopia for as long as possible. I have noticed that older people who take human growth hormone often have a whole or partial reversal of presbyopia.

Reducing stress will also help. The chemicals such as cortisols that are released by the body when we're under stress weaken muscles and diminish the ability of the antioxidants you do have to nourish and protect the eye. See Chapter 6 on cataracts for more detailed advice on nutrients that will protect your vision as you age.

## Your Antioxidant Eye Protection Begins with Glutathione

Before we talk about the nutrients you need in your supplementation program, we want to let you in on some remarkable new discoveries about why these nutrients work. Much is known about the antioxidants we get from food. Many people don't know that our bodies make their own antioxidant substances as well. The names of these are probably unfamiliar to you: Superoxide dismutase, catalase, ubiquinone (more commonly known as coenzyme Q10), and alpha lipoic acid are some that we're discovering have powerful healing abilities. The most plentiful and essential antioxidant our bodies make is called glutathione.

Glutathione is said to be ubiquitous, found in every living cell of every plant, insect, animal, and human. A healthy person's liver produces about 14,000 mg of glutathione a day (about 8½ tsp.), which is carried in the bloodstream to every body cell. To make glutathione, you need sulfur. Foods rich in sulfur include eggs, garlic, onions, and asparagus. You can also get organic sulfur from the supplement MSM, found in your health food store.

Glutathione itself is unstable outside of the body, so the best way to raise its levels with supplements is by taking one of its building blocks, the amino acid cysteine, in the form of N-acetyl cysteine, or NAC.

Your body produces small amounts of a sulfur-rich substance called alpha lipoic acid, which recently has been shown to raise glutathione levels dramatically. You can take alpha lipoic acid in supplement form.

Vitamins C, E, selenium, and beta-carotene all work synergistically with glutathione, re-energizing it as it buffers free radicals throughout the body. The fluid that bathes the lenses of the eyes is especially rich in glutathione and vitamin C.

Low levels of glutathione are found in virtually every disease. University of Michigan researchers recently found that adults who have high glutathione levels are generally healthy, while those with low levels have health problems. By the time surviving subjects were seventy-nine years old, the only ones still alive had high glutathione levels.

What does all this mean? It shows that we should be using glutathione as a marker of health. Glutathione itself is too large a molecule to assimilate well through the digestive tract, so there isn't any good way to supplement it directly, but we can boost the body's production of this powerful antioxidant by eating sulfur-rich foods and taking glutathione-boosting supplements like cysteine and alpha lipoic acid, and other antioxidants such as selenium and vitamins C and E to work with the glutathione.

If you have liver disease, you can take milk thistle (*silymarin*), an herb that boosts glutathione levels in the liver.

## Intravenous Nutrients

Intravenous vitamins and minerals (given via an injection into a vein) can be highly beneficial to your overall health, especially when your health is compromised in some way. We recommend them for a wide range of problems, especially in older people whose ability to absorb nutrients is compromised. In most states, M.D.s or licensed health care professionals working under the direction of an M.D. are the only ones who can legally give injections. If your doctor is interested in learning about giving intravenous vitamins, he or she can find further information in Appendix II at the back of this book.

## Choosing a Multivitamin

A good multivitamin gives you a solid foundation of essential vitamins and minerals. In the upcoming chapters on specific eye diseases, we will name specific nutrients to add to the multivitamin, depending on what eye problems you have. If you are over sixty-five, or if you have difficulty swallowing pills or digesting your food, you may want to use powdered vitamins that are mixed with water or juice. You can get a concentrated dose of nutrients by drinking fresh, organic vegetable juices, too. We make at least one fresh fruit or vegetable juice a day, often combining carrots and celery, or apples and bananas.

No matter who you are or what ailments you have, we recommend that you take a high-potency multivitamin. Here's what you should look for when shopping for one. Most of them require you to take two or three tablets with each meal. Look for a multivitamin that contains the following:

### Beta-carotene/Carotenoids

One-quarter to one-half of beta-carotene taken in is converted to vitamin A, from which your eyes make pigments used for night vision. It's also needed for tissue growth and repair, especially in the mucous membranes of the nose, throat, and lungs. Beta-carotene always should be taken with vitamin E because these two nutrients work together and there is some evidence that beta-carotene can become toxic if taken in high doses alone.

Beta-carotene is found in carrots, leafy greens, yams, and other colorful vegetables and fruits.

Daily dosage: 10,000–15,000 IU

## Vitamin A

The conversion of beta-carotene to vitamin A is not always perfect, so when you have eye disease it pays to take a small amount of vitamin A, too. If your multivitamin doesn't contain vitamin A, you can take it separately. I like the liquid mycel vitamin A. This vitamin can be toxic in high doses over a long period of time, so don't take more than 10,000 IU daily without the supervision of a health care professional.

Daily dosage: 5,000–10,000 IU

## B Vitamins

The B vitamins are essential for the processing of the foods you eat, acting as cogs in the wheel of energy production. They're responsible for maintaining the health of the nervous system and muscle tone. The health of your skin, hair, liver, and eyes suffer if you are deficient in the B vitamins. Food sources are brewer's yeast, meat, and whole-grain cereals. They are also made by the friendly bacteria in your gut.

Here are the daily dosages we recommend for the B vitamins:

Thiamine ($B_1$): 25–50 mg

Riboflavin ($B_2$): 25–100 mg

Niacin (B$_3$): 50–100 mg

Pantothenic acid (B$_5$): 50–100 mg

Pyridoxine (B$_6$): 50–100 mg

Vitamin B$_{12}$: 1,000–2,000 micrograms (mcg)

Biotin: 100–300 mcg

Choline: 50–100 mg

Folic acid (folate or folacin): 200–800 mcg

Inositol: 150–300 mg

## Calcium

More calcium is found in the body than any other mineral. It plays a role in a wide variety of bodily functions. Ninety-nine percent of body calcium is in the bones and teeth, with the remaining percent playing a role in blood clotting, nerve and muscle stimulation, and thyroid gland function. Calcium and magnesium work together to maintain good heart and artery function. The passage of nutrients into and out of cells is reliant on calcium. Natural sources are dairy products, almonds, soybean curd (tofu), broccoli, black-eyed peas, and leafy green vegetables.

Daily dosage: 300–500 mg for men; 600–1,200 mg for women, as calcium citrate, calcium lactate, or calcium gluconate. These are the forms that are best absorbed in the digestive tract.

## *Vitamin D*

You can get vitamin D in two ways: through food or exposure to sunlight. Cholesterol particles in your skin are converted to vitamin D when you go out into the sun. This vitamin aids in the absorption of calcium and the breakdown and assimilation of phosphorus. In other words, it's a crucial bone-building vitamin. It helps make enzymes that carry calcium where it's needed. You don't want to overdo vitamin D in supplement form because, like its fat-soluble cousin vitamin A, it can build up in the tissues and become toxic. Don't take over 400 IU daily without the supervision of a health care professional.

Food sources include cod liver oil and salmon.
Daily dosage: 100–400 IU

## *Vitamin C*

This antioxidant joins forces with vitamins E and beta-carotene to squelch free radicals and prevent oxidation of cholesterol particles. Without a rich supply of vitamin C, blood vessels become weak. People with diets high in vitamin C live longer and suffer less from degenerative diseases like cataracts, macular degeneration, and cancer. Numerous studies have shown its stimulating effect on immune function, which helps your body combat disease with greater strength.

Your need for vitamin C skyrockets when you're sick or stressed. If you can take 2,000 mg of vitamin C daily when you're healthy, you may be able to tolerate 10,000 mg daily when you're sick. Linus Pauling recommended finding out how much vitamin C it takes to give you diarrhea, and then backing off that dose until it goes away.

Foods rich in vitamin C include citrus fruit, mangoes, kiwis, red peppers, and tomatoes.

Daily dosage: 2,000–10,000 mg (2–10 gms)

## Vitamin E

Vitamin E is a powerful fat-soluble antioxidant that re-energizes the other antioxidants and prevents saturated fats and vitamins C and A from becoming oxidized. B vitamins are also protected by vitamin E. Its role in the energy-making machinery of cells in the muscles and heart is an important one and has been studied extensively as a remedy for heart disease. It improves blood flow, decreases the formation of blood clots that can clog blood vessels and cause strokes, strengthens capillary walls, and protects red blood cells and hormones from free radicals. It prevents oxidation of LDL cholesterol, the process believed to be the beginning of unhealthy changes in blood vessel disease.

An important function of vitamin E in the context of eye diseases is that it relieves excessive accumulation of fluid (*edema*), which can be a cause of glaucoma.

Food sources of vitamin E include wheat germ and nuts.

Daily dosage: 400–800 IU, from d-alpha tocopherol

## Boron

This mineral helps keep bones strong.
    Daily dosage: 1–5 mg

## Chromium

This trace mineral is an active ingredient of glucose tolerance factor, which helps your body stay on an even keel with levels of blood sugar and insulin. Fatty acids and cholesterol, both of which your body needs, are synthesized with the help of this mineral. Food sources include brewer's yeast, liver, beef, whole-wheat bread, beets, beet-sugar molasses, and mushrooms. Deficiency is common.
    Daily dosage: 200–400 mcg

## Copper

Copper assists in formation of vital blood components that carry oxygen to your cells. It also is involved in protein metabolism, wound healing, bone and nerve health, and production of elastin (the component of skin that makes it flexible and stretchy). Food sources include liver, whole grains, almonds, green leafy vegetables, dried legumes, and seafood.
    Daily dosage: 1–5 mg

## Magnesium

This mineral makes up a whopping 0.05 percent of your body weight. Seventy percent is located in the bones with calcium and phosphorus, the rest in soft tissues and body fluids. It has so many functions in the body that there are entire medical journals devoted to its study. Evidence is strong that the processed foods prevalent in our diets, as well as mineral depletion from the soil, have left the majority of Americans magnesium deficient. It's needed for normal heart and lung function and energy production from food. Without magnesium, calcium can't work effectively. High blood pressure and weak hearts are improved by intravenous magnesium.

If you are constipated, you can take magnesium that is not chelated—meaning it is not in a citrate, gluconate, or glycinate form—and it will loosen your bowels. Take it in a diluted form in your multivitamin.

Natural food sources of magnesium are almonds and other nuts, raw wheat germ, soy, milk, whole grains, seafood, figs, corn, apples, and seeds.

Daily dosage: 300–500 mg, in the form of magnesium citrate, glycinate, or gluconate. If you have muscle cramps, angina, or osteoporosis, I recommend you take up to 800 mg per day, 400 in the morning and 400 before bed.

### Manganese

Manganese is a trace mineral that helps activate many enzymes needed for use of some of the B vitamins and vitamin C. The synthesis of thyroxine (one of the thyroid hormones), fatty acids, cholesterol, protein, and carbohydrate in the body requires this

mineral. It's also part of skeletal growth, sex hormone formation, and the health of the nervous system. Free radicals cause less damage if they stay
inside the mitochondrion of the cell where they were
formed; manganese keeps them there to be neutral-
ized. Lack of manganese can lead to diabetes and
atherosclerosis.

Food sources of manganese include whole-grain
cereals, egg yolks, nuts, seeds, and green vegetables.

Daily dosage: 10 mg

### Selenium

Selenium is a trace element that has powerful
antioxidant properties. It works with vitamin E to
prevent the oxidation of polyunsaturated fats in the
blood. It is involved in the production of
prostaglandins, important regulatory substances
that keep blood pressure and inflammation under
control. There is evidence that selenium plays a role
in cellular energy production and that it can help
prevent many types of cancer.

Food sources of selenium include brewer's yeast,
organ and muscle meats, fish and shellfish, whole
grains and cereals, and dairy products.

Daily dosage: 25–50 mcg

### Vanadium

This is a trace mineral that helps stabilize blood
sugar.

Daily dosage: 10–25 mcg, as vanadyl sulfate

## Zinc

Zinc's role in alleviating macular degeneration has been thoroughly studied. Zinc deficiency causes deterioration of the macula. This important mineral aids in healing and is a constituent of at least twenty-five enzymes involved in digestion and metabolism. It helps vitamin A to be released from the liver so it can be used in eye tissues.

Food sources of zinc include whole grains, brewer's yeast, wheat bran, wheat germ, and pumpkin seeds.

Daily dosage: 10–30 mg

We can't emphasize enough that the health of your whole body, particularly of your blood vessels, will be the key to improving your vision. The doses of nutrients already in your multivitamin, combined with the recommended dosages in the chapters that follow on specific eye diseases, might require you to take extra pills.

Bring this book to your health food store and have the vitamin clerk help you choose the best combination of supplements at the best price. There are supplements on the market now that are designed for eye problems and that can make it easier and more economical to follow these recommendations. You'll find information in Appendix II about mail-order supplements if you can't find them locally.

One way to avoid taking too many pills is to take a multivitamin low in the bulky nutrients. You can take vitamin C separately, as well as a separate calcium/magnesium supplement, all of which add a lot of bulk to multivitamins.

**IN SHORT . . .**

1.  Avoid simple carbohydrates like sugar
    and white-flour products. Eat complex
    carbohydrates in moderation and with a
    balanced amount of protein and fat.
    When you do have a sweet treat, make
    it a healthy one. If you are diabetic, be
    especially wary of refined carbohy-
    drates.

2.  Cook with olive or canola oil. Avoid
    hydrogenated oils and chips, cookies,
    and other baked goods that contain
    them. A pat of butter on your toast is
    okay, as long as you practice modera-
    tion when it comes to fat intake. Limit
    fat calories to 25–30 percent of your
    calories.

3.  For most people, high levels of choles-
    terol in the blood are a symptom, not a
    cause, of disease. Worry less about
    altering your total cholesterol and more
    about living healthfully. Try to wean
    yourself off cholesterol-lowering drugs
    with the guidance of your physician.
    (Never stop a drug abruptly.) Pay more
    attention to reducing stress, keeping
    antioxidant levels high, avoiding harm-
    ful fats, and limiting exposure to toxins.

4.  Eat whole, unprocessed foods made
    from ingredients you recognize. Buy
    organic whenever possible.

5. Nutritional supplements added to a healthy diet keep your eyes (and the rest of you) functioning at their best!
6. If you have eye disease, take the nutritional prescription recommended daily, without fail.

## YOUR MULTIVITAMIN SHOULD INCLUDE . . .

Beta-carotene/carotenoids: 10,000–15,000 IU

Vitamin A: 5,000–10,000 IU

The B vitamins:

Thiamine ($B_1$): 25–50 mg

Riboflavin ($B_2$): 25–100 mg

Niacin ($B_3$): 50–100 mg

Pantothenic acid ($B_5$): 50–100 mg

Pyridoxine ($B_6$): 50–100 mg

Vitamin $B_{12}$: 1,000–2,000 micrograms (mcg)

Biotin: 100–300 mcg

Choline: 50–100 mg

Folic acid : 400–800 mcg

Inositol: 150–300 mg

Calcium: 300–500 mg for men; 600–1,200 mg for women

Vitamin D: 100–400 IU

Vitamin C: 2,000–10,000 mg (2–10 g)

Vitamin E: 400–800 IU

Boron: 1–5 mg
Chromium: 200–400 mcg
Copper: 1–5 mg
Magnesium: 300–500 mg, and up to 800
    mg for specific health problems
Manganese: 10 mg
Selenium: 25–50 mcg
Vanadyl sulfate: 10–25 mcg
Zinc: 10–30 mg

# 4

# Preventing and Healing Macular Degeneration

Age-related macular degeneration is the most common cause of blindness in Americans over the age of fifty. Up to fifteen million people who fall into this age group are affected. Up to 10 percent of senior citizens in the seventh decade of life have vision loss from macular degeneration. Between the ages of seventy-five and eighty-five, up to 28 percent of Americans will lose some central vision due to age-related macular degeneration (ARMD). It is the fastest-growing cause of legal blindness in the United States.

If you are over sixty-five, if you have blue, green, or hazel eyes (brown eyes have more protective melanin pigment over the retina), if you have been frequently exposed to sunlight, especially without protective eyewear, if you are a smoker, or if you are a postmenopausal woman, you are more likely to develop this disease.

For such a prevalent problem, there is very little that mainstream medicine can do to stop its progression towards total central blindness.

## How the Eye Is Damaged in
## Macular Degeneration

Within the eye is a layer filled with tiny blood vessels (choroidal capillaries) that nourish the retina. In people who make poor diet and lifestyle choices over the years, these capillaries become clogged with calcium deposits and cholesterol. Oxygen can't reach the retina and the cells starve and die.

In other instances, the capillary lining (endothelium) may become weakened, allowing fluid and blood components to escape where they shouldn't. The result is increased pressure in the area of the retina, which can cause death of retinal cells.

The role of oxidation in this process is complex. It plays a part in the blood vessel diseases that lead to clogged capillaries, arteries, and veins. Lack of antioxidants in the diet allows free radicals to run rampant, and this process carries much of the responsibility for the vessels becoming blocked in the first place. (Refer to Chapter 10, where we discuss the circulatory system in detail.)

Once blood flow to the retina is reduced or cut off, the natural antioxidant defenses of the body that are carried in the blood can't counter the sunlight-caused oxidative damage going on in the retina, and deterioration is accelerated.

The retinal pigment epithelium (RPE) is a single cell layer that brings nutrients and oxygen into the retina, flushing wastes into the bloodstream. The aging spots (drusen) that often occur in macular degeneration appear on the RPE. Thirty percent of adults have drusen, and in many no visual impairment results, so the deterioration may go unnoticed. But meanwhile, the macular degeneration can continue to progress.

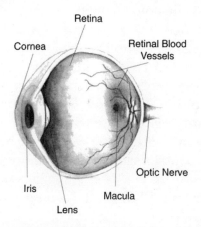

Macular degeneration occurs in and around the retinal blood vessels that surround the macula.

Calcium deposits also can build up in the membrane that lies between the choroidal capillary layer and the RPE. This blocks exchange of blood, nutrients, and wastes, threatening the health of the retina.

A substance called lipofuscin, which is hardened vitamin A that has been used and discarded by the retinal cells, also can accumulate in the RPE, clogging normal cell metabolism. This process is the result of passing years. Lipofuscin plays a key role in the production of harmful free radicals and leads to lipid peroxidation ("tagging" of blood-borne fat molecules by free radicals, rendering them dangerous to your cells). Overexposure to ultraviolet and (especially) blue light is the first step in lipofuscin's generation of free radicals.

A layer of nerves links the retina to the optic nerve. Within this layer are protective pigments that are yellow in color, called *lutein* and *zeaxanthin*. These are members of the group of antioxidant substances known as *carotenoids,* found in colorful vegetables and fruits. Green, leafy vegetables like spinach, kale, and collard greens are rich in lutein and zeaxanthin. In a study of 870 people aged fifty-five to eighty years, those who ate spinach or collard greens two to four times a week were half as likely to develop macular degeneration as those who ate them once a month or less. These pigments provide a blue-light "sunglass" filter for the central retina.

---

### VEGETABLES RICH IN LUTEIN AND ZEAXANTHIN

Spinach
Mustard greens
Kale
Broccoli
Parsley
Celery
Green peas
Brussels sprouts
Pumpkin
Squash
Carrots
Yams
Corn
Green beans

# Early Detection of Macular Degeneration

Macular degeneration develops very slowly, and the time to catch it is in the early stages. Even better, take steps to *prevent* it altogether early in life. The more advanced the disease, the harder you'll have to work to make progress in halting it.

### SYMPTOMS OF MACULAR DEGENERATION

Normally straight objects appear bent or wavy.

A dark, blank or blurry spot appears in the center of your vision.

When you cover up one eye, what you're looking at changes size or color.

Charlie, a fisherman, is a good example. He came to our clinic to have his eyes checked for the first time in his life.

"I can't see to drive anymore, especially at night," he told me. "I'm having trouble reading. Guess it's come time for me to get some glasses." Charlie loves his work, and when he's not out on the water casting his nets, he's at the harbor doing repairs on his boat. He's not planning to retire any time soon, although he's almost seventy, and he gets plenty of exercise. His dark tan gives him a look of good health. His smoking habit has lasted fifty-five years, and he doesn't have much desire to quit now. "I'm gettin' too old to be depriving myself of the little pleasures," he said as I made a few notes in his chart.

I asked Charlie exactly how his vision had changed over the past few months. "It's real odd," he said, his pale blue eyes crinkling at the corners. "The outlines of things are sorta wavy. Things that oughta be straight seem to be bent in the middle. I'm having trouble seeing people's faces, even. The other day my grandson came by the harbor where I was working, and I didn't recognize him. Now my daughter's worried I'm senile, but I just couldn't make out his face." He thought a moment. "Oh, also, when I go below from outside in the sun, I'm practically blind for a good minute or two before my eyes get used to the dark. I end up tripping all over the place down there."

A diagnosis of early macular degeneration wasn't hard to make in Charlie's case. When I looked at his retinas I saw patches of drusen, age spots much like those that appear on the skin of people often exposed to the sun. Charlie also was tested with a copy of the Amsler grid, which looks like a piece of graph paper with a dot at its center. I asked Charlie to look at the central dot and to tell me whether the lines began to seem wavy. "Well, yeah, now that you mention it," he murmured. "That's some neat trick!" Not surprisingly, Charlie had never heard of the disease I had diagnosed him with.

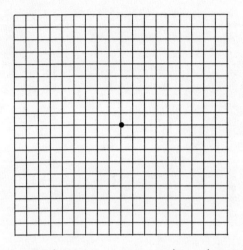

The Amsler Grid: Wearing your reading glasses, cover one eye, and focus on the dot in the middle of the grid above. Then repeat the test for the other eye. In healthy eyes, all of the lines are straight, and the squares are the same size. If there is any distortion, as in the diagram below, you may have macular degeneration.

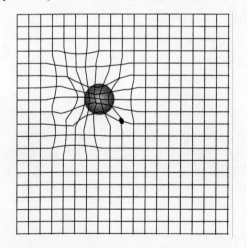

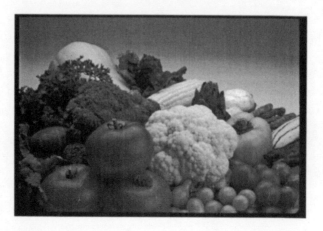

Blurring at the center of vision may be a symptom of macular degeneration.

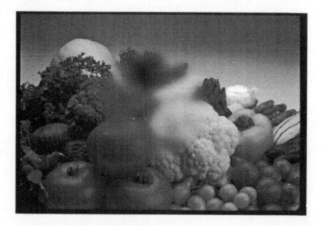

## How Macular Degeneration Gets Started and Develops

Macular degeneration takes years to develop, and vision loss can be very subtle in its earlier stages. The affected part of the eye lies in a pit only 2 mm wide in the center of the retina. The retina, which is a paper-thin, postage-stamp-sized area on the inside back portion of the eyeball, is the part of the eye that does the miraculous and delicate work of translating light energy into nerve impulses. These impulses travel from the eye to the brain along the optic nerve, and the brain then translates the message from the nerve into a picture of what you're looking at.

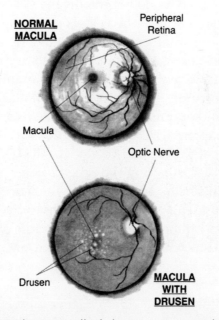

Age spots on the eye called drusen are an early sign of macular degeneration.

There are two kinds of macular degeneration. The dry (nonexudative) form is much more common, less severe, and rarely causes blindness, but can become the more dangerous, wet (exudative) form at any time.

The dry form of macular degeneration can consist of either poor circulation in the tiny blood vessels of the eye, or damaged blood vessels that create scar tissue and new blood vessel growth that blocks vision.

Blood seeping out of the retinal vessels *(hemorrhage)* is one characteristic of wet macular degeneration. The increased fluid pressure caused by hemorrhage damages the macula. The wet form also can involve growth of new blood vessels to replace clogged ones. The body's intelligence is counterproductive here because the vessels grow over the macula, causing total central blindness. Even in this most severe form of macular degeneration, all sight is not lost; some peripheral vision is maintained.

Careful food and supplement choices can help you to avoid or diminish these problems, as you'll see in this chapter.

Much of the advice we give to ARMD patients is geared towards halting the progression and preventing the shift from the dry form, which doesn't usually cause total loss of central vision, to the wet form, which does. In neither form is there loss of peripheral vision, but when the disease is advanced, it's still nearly impossible to move around normally, read, watch TV, or identify people.

We think that macular degeneration is caused by a combination of oxidation damage and the consequences of poor circulation. Your retinal cells are especially vulnerable to oxidation because they are exposed to ultraviolet radiation.

Human eyes contain a dark pigment called melanin, designed to prevent back reflection of light. It also serves as a shield from ultraviolet radiation. Those with light-colored eyes don't have as much melanin pigment at the back of their eyes as do dark-eyed people; this explains why dark-eyed people are less likely to have ARMD. No matter what your eye color, melanin begins to deteriorate by the age of fifty, and that's when macular degeneration develops in earnest.

The macula is right at the focal point of light's entry into the eye. People who work outdoors without proper eye protection, like our friend Charlie, show signs of macular degeneration more often and earlier in life than those who spend much of their time indoors.

Within your eyes, protective shields of vitamin E and carotenoids (both of which are antioxidants, derived from the foods you eat) work to balance free radicals, staving off sun damage. Macular disease usually starts near the edge of the macula, where antioxidant protection is weakest and where daily bombardment by solar radiation first takes its toll.

## Mainstream Treatments for Macular Degeneration

Taking good care of yourself physically, emotionally, mentally, and spiritually is your foundation for everlasting vision, but there are still times when surgery and other mainstream interventions are necessary. We perform eye surgery in our clinics every day, and the patients who do best are those who take care of themselves on every level.

If your ophthalmologist recommends these procedures or drugs, you will know what to expect and you will be able to make educated choices about your treatment.

For the dry form of macular degeneration, there is no mainstream medical treatment. Ninety percent of macular degeneration sufferers have the dry form. This means that they have some deterioration of the retinal cells responsible for central vision, but little or no growth of new blood vessels over the central retina (macula).

## Laser Treatment

For those who have the wet form of macular degeneration, laser treatment *(photocoagulation)* can be used to stop the growth of these sight-threatening new blood vessels. A tiny laser beam is aimed at leaks in blood vessels, and when it hits them, it seals them shut. This procedure doesn't restore vision or permanently arrest the progression of the disease. It is a temporary stopgap measure. Laser treatment can actually destroy retinal tissues and impair vision even more. Because it isn't a permanent solution, repeated treatments are required, and with each treatment more retinal tissues are damaged by the treatment itself. We want to emphasize that laser surgery works only for those with the advanced *wet* form of this disease. Once new blood vessels have begun to grow, nutritional therapy becomes much less effective, and your choices are limited to drugs, surgery, or radiation treatments.

The worse your vision is to start with, the better your chances for improvement with laser surgery. Very few people with macular degeneration meet the eligibility criteria for laser surgery. Look at it as a last resort.

We recommend that all but the most severe macular disease patients postpone laser treatment until they've tried the preventive and restorative options found in this book for six to nine months. If your eye doctor suggests laser treatments, be sure to ask her or him the following questions:

✓ What percentage of your patients have kept their vision for five years after laser treatment?

✓ Would you have laser treatment if you were in my position?

✓ Can you tell me about any cases where vision has actually improved following laser surgery?

✓ Will you read the surgical consent form out loud to me and explain any details I don't understand?

## Radiation Treatment

Ionizing radiation, the same kind used in the treatment of cancer, has also been used in the treatment of wet macular degeneration. The drawbacks of this method are much the same as those of laser treatment: The "cure" may do more damage than the disease. Preservation of remaining vision is the aim with most of these mainstream treatments; they don't bring back vision that's been lost. The adverse effects of exposure to radiation are well known: It works by killing unwanted cells, but often takes healthy tissues with the unhealthy ones. In this way it can delay the growth of new blood vessels over the retina. This is another last-resort treatment for advanced disease where there is significant central vision loss.

## Photodynamic Therapy

A new experimental treatment called *photodynamic therapy* is being studied. Using special molecules that make cells more sensitive to light, surgeons purposely cause the production of free radicals. They try to do so only in diseased tissues, so that the body's natural oxidation process can do the job of destroying unwanted blood vessel growth. Photodynamic therapy is also meant only for the treatment of advanced macular degeneration.

## Anti-angiogenesis Drugs

Another emerging mainstream therapy for those with wet macular degeneration is *anti-angiogenesis* (*angio* means "blood vessels" and *genesis* means "creation" or "formation"). This treatment uses drugs to prevent the new blood vessel growth that occurs in the wet form of macular degeneration. Thalidomide, the drug given to pregnant women in the sixties that caused severe birth defects in thousands of children, is now being used as an anti-angiogenesis drug. So far it's been shown to be safe for this type of treatment, but it is very expensive and its effectiveness is as yet unproven.

Interferon is another anti-angiogenesis drug. Its value in the treatment of wet macular degeneration has not been shown convincingly, and there are major side effects. Some researchers think it holds promise as a companion treatment to laser surgery. In one study, 18 percent of those treated with interferon had to discontinue the drug because of severe adverse reactions. Flu-like symptoms including fever, headaches, muscles aches, and chills affect almost half of those treated with interferon.

## Stay Away from Aspirin

The blood-thinning action of aspirin has led some eye doctors to recommend it for improving blood flow to the retinas of those with either form of macular degeneration, but some studies have shown that aspirin actually can cause macular degeneration by creating retinal hemorrhages (tiny leaks in the blood vessels of the retina). Other nonsteroidal anti-inflammatory drugs (NSAIDs) such as ibuprofen can cause tiny retinal hemorrhages in healthy eyes. Those with macular degeneration have very delicate eye vessels and often also have high blood pressure. Both factors predispose them to retinal hemorrhages, which will only be aggravated by NSAIDs. Aspirin and other NSAIDs are also damaging to the delicate lining of the gastrointestinal tract.

The bottom line is that although aspirin may help prevent blood clots and improve blood flow to the retina, the risks seem to outweigh the benefits in those with eye disease. There are plenty of natural ways to improve blood flow to the retina that are without risk. For example, nutrients with anti-inflammatory action include omega-3 and omega-6 fatty acids, garlic, magnesium, and vitamin E.

## Transplanting Retinal Cells

Some exciting work is being done with transplantation of healthy retinal cells to replace damaged ones. This procedure may be available to people with macular diseases at some time in the next few years, although it's too early to tell whether retinal cell transplantation will be the long-sought cure for macular degeneration. In the meantime, there's plenty you can do to maintain your remaining vision.

Lasers, radiation, and anti-angiogenesis drugs are used to treat the wet form of macular degeneration. This severe form, which can rapidly cause blindness, sometimes calls for drastic treatment measures. This is the reason we strongly recommend that you implement the lifestyle and nutritional changes suggested in this book to help you *prevent* the transformation from dry to wet macular degeneration. Other therapies are recommended only when all else has failed to help.

# Nutritional Prescription for Macular Degeneration

### Vitamin C and Bioflavonoids

Taking extra vitamin C when you have the dry form of macular degeneration helps prevent broken blood vessels and new blood vessel growth across the macula.

Bioflavonoids, which are packaged with vitamin C in nature and enhance the action of vitamin C, are found in colorful fruits such as berries, lemons, grapes, plums, black currants, grapefruit, apricots, and cherries. Rose hips are a popular source of bioflavonoids used in vitamin C supplements.

Essential for proper absorption and use of vitamin C, bioflavonoids assist in maintaining the intercellular glue (collagen) that strengthens connective tissue throughout the body. They have antioxidant powers and are essential for strong blood vessels. As supplements, you can buy quercetin or extract of ginkgo biloba, bilberry, grapeseed, or cranberry. Bilberry specifically goes to the eyes and improves night vision.

Daily dosage: at least 2,000 mg of vitamin C, and 200–400 mg of bioflavonoids

## Beta-carotene and Vitamin A

It pays to load up on beta-carotene, which is harmless in high doses as long as it's taken with vitamin E. I recommend you also take vitamin A, in case your body isn't converting the beta-carotene properly.

Daily dosage: beta-carotene, 15,000–25,000 IU

Daily dosage: vitamin A, 10,000–25,000 IU (no more than 10,000 if you are pregnant or could become pregnant)

## Lutein and Zeaxanthin

Within the nerve layer of the eye, these protective yellow carotenoid pigments work as a blue-light sun filter for the central retina. Until recently, the importance of lutein was largely overlooked by researchers. A study published in the *Journal of the American Medical Association* showed that adults who regularly consume spinach and collard greens are much less likely to have macular degeneration. Since the three highest-risk groups for macular degeneration—smokers, postmenopausal women, and adults with light-colored eyes—all have half as much lutein and zeaxanthin at the back of their eyes, it's assumed that these pigments have something to do with the disease.

A few weeks after consuming more lutein-rich foods or lutein supplements, some normal-sighted people report less glare, improved color vision, and sharper vision.

Whether you're eating lutein-rich foods or using the supplements, try not to do so at the same meal during which you're taking a beta-carotene supplement or eating beta-carotene-rich foods. They compete for absorption in the digestive tract and for transport on cholesterol particles from the liver to the eye.

Spinach, collard greens, and kale are good food sources. Supplements are derived from marigold flower petals.

Daily dosage: 6–10 mg of lutein, 0.3–1 mg of zeaxanthin

## *Magnesium*

This important mineral works as a natural chelator by playing a key role in the absorption and metabolism of calcium. It is essential to the proper functioning of the heart, and acts as a co-factor for hundreds of biochemical actions in the body. It aids blood flow to the eyes by maintaining proper fluid balance in the cells and reducing muscle spasms.

Daily dosage: 300–500 mg at bedtime

## *Cold-water Fish and Fish Oils*

A serving of cold-water fish such as salmon, tuna, cod, mackerel, or sardines is rich in vitamins A and D. The vitamin A found in these fish is absorbed and used by the body more easily than beta-carotene. Excess is stored in the liver and can be accessed when the eyes need to make more of the visual pigment needed for sight. The consequences of vitamin A and beta-carotene deficiency are seen commonly in developing countries. The rate of blindness in children is much higher, and adults suffer more from an eye disease known as *keratomalacia,* which begins with night blindness and progresses to blindness.

Fish oils are also superior sources of the essential oils known as omega-3 fatty acids. These fatty acids have been studied extensively for their positive effects on cardiovascular diseases and related problems.

Decreased blood clotting is a proven benefit gained by people who eat plenty of fish. Anything that helps keep blood vessels clear helps keep macular degeneration from progressing. Diets deficient in omega-3 oils have been shown to result in visual impairment in animal studies.

Because omega-3 oils are unsaturated, they easily can become rancid, which is the down side of taking them in supplement form. If they are rancid, they will do you more harm than good. Our preference is that you eat cold-water fish at least twice a week, but if you absolutely can't stand fish, go ahead and take a supplement. Look for a brand that specifies that the oil has been preserved in some way, then break open a capsule and smell it to be sure it's not rancid. Take the capsules with meals. If you're burping up fish oil, a truly unpleasant experience, that may be an indication that the supplements are rancid or you're taking too much.

Daily dosage: Follow the directions on the container

### Vitamin E

Taking vitamin E every day will keep oxidation at bay and keep blood vessels to the eyes healthy. Alpha tocopherol, a form of vitamin E, is found distributed across the retina; where it is sparse is where the early signs of macular degeneration occur.

Daily dosage: 800 IU

## Selenium

Selenium is a component of glutathione peroxidase, which protects cell membranes from oxidation. It also has potent antiviral effects.

Daily dosage: at least 200 mcg

## N-acetyl cysteine (NAC)

Take this to keep your glutathione levels high.

Daily dosage: 500 mg, 2–3 times

## Taurine

This amino acid is important to good eye and blood vessel health.

Daily dosage: 500–2,000 mg between meals

## Garlic

This flavorful bulb will keep blood from clotting, raise HDL, and lower LDL. If you don't include fresh, raw garlic (the best kind) in your food on a near-daily basis because you don't like the odor, try odorless garlic capsules. If you like the flavor and don't mind the odor, use it plentifully. It's also high in sulfur, which will encourage the production of glutathione.

Daily dosage: about 1,000 mg of the odorless capsules

### Zinc

This helps release vitamin A from the liver.

Daily dosage: 15–30 mg if your multivitamin is low in zinc

### Coenzyme Q10

This powerful antioxidant will energize the heart and improve circulation.

Daily dosage: 30–200 mg

### Hydrochloric Acid

If you don't have enough stomach acid (see Chapter 9 on digestion), a supplement can help.

Daily dosage: 250 mg beta hydrochloride, with meals

IN SHORT . . .

1.  Age-related macular degeneration is the most common cause of legal blindness in Americans over the age of fifty.

2.  While central vision can deteriorate badly, those with macular degeneration do not go completely blind. They maintain some peripheral vision, no matter how advanced the disease.

3.  If you are over sixty-five, have light-colored eyes with little protective melanin pigment, often have been exposed to sunlight without protective eyewear, are or have been a smoker, or are a postmenopausal female, you are at greater risk for this disease than the general population.

4.  Symptoms include decreased night vision, trouble making the adjustment from light to dark environments, difficulty recognizing faces, and difficulty reading, writing, and driving. Objects that should be straight will appear to have a bend in the middle. Your ophthalmologist can make a diagnosis using an Amsler grid and by checking for drusen (age spots) on the back of the eye.

5.  The dry form of macular degeneration is the most common and is best controlled by diet and supplements. In this

form, there is some deterioration of retinal cells, but no hemorrhage or growth of new blood vessels. Vision loss may be minimal if the progression from the dry to the wet form is stopped by using the advice in these pages. The wet form involves leakage of blood into the vitreous humor that fills the eyeball and also the growth of new blood vessels across the retina.

6. Lasers, interferon, and thalidomide are the mainstream treatments of choice. These are used only in treatment of the wet form of the disease and don't often have good results. Retinal cell transplants may be possible in the next few years.

7. A summary of the nutritional "Rx" for macular degeneration can be found in Appendix I at the end of this book.

# 5

# Preventing and Healing Glaucoma

Nicknamed "the sneak thief of sight," glaucoma is the most common cause of blindness in the United States. It is especially insidious because it can progress to an advanced stage before sight is lost. Except for one rare type of glaucoma, there is no sensation of pain as it encroaches upon the delicate optic nerve. Because it is side vision that is affected, glaucoma often goes unnoticed until a significant amount of vision is lost. Even eye doctors have trouble making a diagnosis of this disease.

Glaucoma is most often a disease associated with aging. According to the National Society for the Prevention of Blindness, as many as three out of one hundred Americans over age sixty-five have glaucoma. You are at a higher risk for glaucoma if you have diabetes or a family history of glaucoma.

There are several kinds of glaucoma. All of them involve damage to the optic nerve, the passageway for visual information into the brain. How the damage comes about results in the differences between them.

Within your eyeballs is a fluid called the aqueous humor that gives the eyeball its shape and resiliency. Your eyes make this fluid, and there is a fluid drain within the eye so that any excess can be removed. Just as blood pressure fluctuates depending on activity, diet, and emotions, so does the fluid pressure within the eyes. It's all controlled by a delicate regulatory system. If this system gets out of balance, eye pressure can be elevated chronically, just as blood pressure can. Under this pressure the optic nerve is literally squashed by the pressure of the aqueous humor around it. Increased pressure on the optic nerve results in death of its cells from the outside in towards the center. The gradual deterioration of vision creates tunnel vision—the opposite of what happens in macular degeneration.

## Diagnosing Glaucoma

While glaucoma has been intensely studied, it has been very difficult for researchers to come to an agreement on how to diagnose it. High fluid pressure within the eye *(intraocular pressure)* is a well-established cause of the most common variety of glaucoma and is treated aggressively when diagnosed. Risk of glaucoma increases with increasing intraocular pressure, but a diagnosis of elevated eye pressure is not the same thing as a diagnosis of glaucoma.

In people with raised eye pressure, optic disc

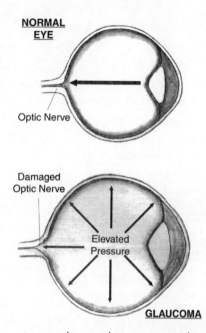

**NORMAL EYE**

Optic Nerve

Damaged Optic Nerve

Elevated Pressure

**GLAUCOMA**

Glaucoma can cause elevated pressure within the eye
that causes permanent damage to the optic nerve

changes, and vision loss, the diagnosis of glaucoma
is unquestionable. The problem is that some eye
physicians will make a diagnosis based solely on eye
pressure measurements, assuming that elevated
pressure on the optic nerve will *inevitably* cause
damage and vision loss if left untreated. That is not
always the case. Some people with high eye pressure
don't lose any significant amount of peripheral
vision. Some people with normal or even low eye
pressure have glaucoma.

Treatment of glaucoma and elevated eye fluid

pressure (also known as *ocular hypertension*) with various drugs, which is the typical route taken by mainstream eye doctors, may end up doing the patient more harm than good. Not only can the drugs be harmful, they also don't do much to preserve vision in those who are suffering from glaucoma. It's important to be sure you actually have glaucoma before taking the drugs, since they do have negative side effects.

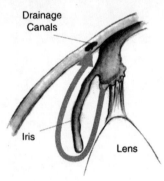

In open-angle glaucoma the drainage canals for eye fluid may be blocked.

## Types of Glaucoma

### 1. Simple or Chronic Open-Angle Glaucoma

In this type of glaucoma, the fluid drain is not totally stopped up but clogged. Fluid is coming into your eyes but isn't draining out efficiently, which increases the pressure inside the eye. If you have clogged arteries, high blood pressure, or diabetes; if you

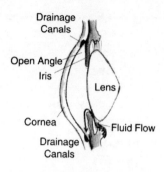

Open-Angle Glaucoma

smoke or drink to excess; if you are of African ancestry; or if you have a history of severe anemia or shock—you are at a higher risk for open-angle glaucoma. This is by far the most common type of glaucoma, representing 70 to 90 percent of glaucoma cases.

This is the true "sneak thief of the night" type of glaucoma, because it can progress very slowly over many years, and by the time it's noticed, much vision already may be permanently destroyed.

## 2. Closed-Angle Glaucoma

When the fluid drains within the eyes are completely blocked, closed-angle glaucoma results. What could block the eye's drain canals? Some people are genetically predisposed to this kind of glaucoma because of the shape of their eyes. In other cases, the lens of the eye may bulge too far forward, or the iris pigment layer thickens and closes the fluid drain when the pupil dilates in response to light.

## Secondary Closed-Angle Glaucoma

Secondary glaucoma is brought on by a known factor. For example, steroid medications, often prescribed for asthma or for healing after eye surgery, cause changes in the molecules within the eye drain and cause it to swell shut (steroid-induced glaucoma). Flakes of pigment may come off the iris (pigmentary glaucoma) or particles may flake from the lens (pseudoexfoliative glaucoma) and become lodged in the drain. Allergies may cause the drain to become blocked by release of histamine (allergic glaucoma).

## Acute Closed-Angle Glaucoma

Most glaucoma of the closed-angle type is chronic, meaning it takes a long time to come on, and its progression is gradual. But sometimes, in acute glaucoma, the eye pressure rises suddenly, causing severe pain, nausea, and even vomiting. This type of glaucoma causes intense pain and requires immediate laser surgery to open a path for the eye fluid. Until that happens, unwanted pressures are exerted on the optic nerve and may cause permanent damage. Acute glaucoma can be caused by eye drops that dilate the pupil or anticholinergic medications such as Donnatol (commonly prescribed for stomach cramps).

### *3. Low-Pressure or Low-Tension Glaucoma (also known as Circulatory Glaucoma)*

In this type of glaucoma, eye pressure is well within normal ranges and sometimes goes below normal.

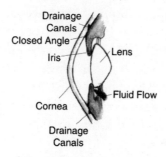

Closed-Angle Glaucoma

The only symptom is loss of side vision. Circulatory glaucoma is the result of poor circulation to the eyes. This often reflects a weak heart muscle that can't pump enough blood to the extremities. Even if the heart is strong, constriction of blood vessels *(vasospasm)* caused by stress, high blood cholesterol levels, an imbalance of calcium and magnesium, or a combination of all three, can keep blood away from the optic nerve. Those who have this type of glaucoma usually suffer from heart disease as well. Optic nerve cells die for lack of nutrients and oxygen, resulting in vision loss.

## 4. Toxic Glaucoma, or Toxic Optic Neuropathy

Toxic glaucoma is a type of secondary glaucoma because it is brought on by known substances that are toxic to eye nerve cells. Cigarette smoke, the flavor enhancer monosodium glutamate (MSG), and (in some sensitive people) aspartame are all optic nerve toxins. Glutamate is a neurotransmitter and a crucial dietary component, but if levels climb too high, it becomes harmful to your body.

You may think that MSG, a compound very high in glutamate, is found only in Chinese restaurant food, but it is everywhere these days. It is nearly always found in foods served in restaurants and is used in thousands of packaged foods, including most so-called health foods. Packaged foods designed for children tend to be especially high in MSG. At least twenty different names are used on food labels to disguise MSG. (See the box "The Many Disguises of MSG," below.) Ask the server at your favorite restaurants to have the chef omit the MSG from your meal.

Aspartame, commonly known as NutraSweet, is not a well-understood substance and has been linked to loss of memory and headaches. I'd advise you to avoid it if at all possible.

 THE MANY DISGUISES OF MSG

The packaged food industry has gotten very clever about disguising the presence of MSG in its food. Read labels carefully.

**Additives That Always Contain MSG (Monosodium Glutamate):**

Hydrolyzed Vegetable Protein
Hydrolyzed Protein
Hydrolyzed Plant Protein
Plant Protein Extract
Sodium Caseinate
Calcium Caseinate

Yeast Extract
Textured Protein
Autolyzed Yeast
Hydrolyzed Oat Flour

**Additives That Frequently Contain MSG:**
Malt Extract
Malt Flavoring
Bouillon
Broth Stock
Flavoring
Natural Flavoring
Natural Beef or Chicken Flavoring
Seasoning
Spices

**Additives That *May* Contain MSG or Excitotoxins:**
Carrageenan
Enzymes
Soy Protein Concentrate
Soy Protein Isolate
Whey Protein Isolate

Reprinted with permission from *Excitotoxins: The Taste That Kills,* by Russell L. Blaylock, M.D., (1997). Health Press, Santa Fe, N.M.

## Steroid-Induced Glaucoma

This is a form of toxic glaucoma brought on by long-term use of oral or inhaled steroid medications such as those prescribed for asthma. Even steroid skin creams, used over long periods, are absorbed into the system sufficiently to act as an optic nerve toxin. Steroid drugs rob the body of vitamin C, and the concentration of this antioxidant in the eyes is many times higher than in the rest of the body. Chronically high stress levels have the same effect on vitamin C levels; this makes sense, because the body's stress hormones are steroids and have the same (although less intense) action as steroid drugs. Use the natural anti-inflammatory measures I describe throughout this book.

## Glaucoma Caused by Inflammation or Malnutrition

Eye infections such as those caused by herpes or other viruses, or in chronic inflammatory conditions, mean increased risk of glaucoma. What do you think most doctors will prescribe to control inflammation in the eye? Ironically, steroids, which, as you know by now, can *cause* glaucoma.

Malnutrition, poor absorption of crucial nutrients through the walls of the intestines, and pernicious anemia (usually caused by problems making or absorbing the vitamin $B_{12}$ and often treated with $B_{12}$ injections) also can lead to optic nerve damage and vision loss.

# Mainstream Treatments for Glaucoma

## Drugs Used to Treat Glaucoma

Drugs designed to relieve fluid pressure around the optic nerve make up the conventional treatment plan for this disease. If you have primary open-angle glaucoma or ocular hypertension, your eye doctor will probably prescribe one or more of the following medications:

## Beta-blocker Eye Drops

Beta-blocker eye drops (Levobunolol, AKBeta, Betagan Liquifilm, Betoptic, OptiPranolol, Ocupress, Timolol, Betimol, Timoptic) decrease pressure by slowing the production of fluid in the eye. Side effects are common with any beta-blocker drug. You may experience depression, decreased sex drive, lowered heart rate, balance loss, or breathing problems while using this medication. It should not be used by people with asthma or by those who are already taking beta-blockers orally to treat other conditions. It's crucial that you use only the dose prescribed; more isn't better in this instance.

Apraclonidine HCl (Iopidine), an alpha-agonist eye drop that has the same pressure-lowering effect as the beta-blockers, is often used in addition to other medications if they are not sufficiently reducing eye pressure. Often it is prescribed to counteract the rise in eye pressure that can occur after eye surgery. A new alpha-agonist eye drop is brimonidine tartrate (Alphagan).

## Epinephrine/Sympathomimetic Eye Drops

Epinephrine/sympathomimetic eye drops (Glaucon, Epinephrine HCl, Epifrin, Epinal) increase outflow

through the fluid drain of the eye. Epinephrine causes stinging and burning when used, and vision may
be blurry for a while after instillation. It should be
used with caution in those with history of high blood
pressure, diabetes, overactive thyroid gland, heart
disease, stroke, or asthma. These drops can cause
your blood pressure to shoot up, heart rate to speed
up or become irregular, or may bring on anginal
pains in susceptible people. Some people feel light-
headed or faint when using these eye drops. Long-
term use can lead to pigment deposits on the cornea
and in the eye membranes (conjunctiva). If the drops
become discolored or separated, you should throw
them away. We don't recommend these drugs
because of their dangerous side effects. There are
other more effective and safer drugs available.

Dipivefrin HCl (Propine, AKPro) is a substance
that turns into epinephrine when dropped into the
eye. The side effects are milder and it should be used
by those with risk for dangerous side effects with epinephrine. Rise in blood pressure and rapid or irregular heartbeat can occur with this medication as
well, but there is much less stinging with these
drops.

## Miotics/Parasympathomimetic Eye Drops

Miotics/parasympathomimetic eye drops (carbachol,
pilocarpine, or combinations of these; there are
dozens of brand names) also work to increase outflow of fluid from the eye. They have fewer side
effects than other pressure-relieving eye drops.

These medications work by stimulating the muscles that change the dimensions of the lens. Resistance to outflow of fluid is reduced.

These drugs are inappropriate for some forms of secondary glaucoma and are not advisable for those who have ulcers, hyperthyroidism, cramps in the digestive tract, urinary tract obstruction, Parkinson's disease, recent heart attack, or high or low blood pressure. In some people they can cause retinal detachment; be certain that your eye doctor checks to see if you are at risk for this problem before you start with miotics. When using these medications, use caution while driving at night or performing any task in dim light because they can adversely affect your ability to adjust to dark environments.

There are two main categories of miotic eye drops: pilocarpine and carbachol. All may sting when drops are put into the eyes, can cause headache or browache, decrease night vision, and should not be used by those who have asthma. Systemic side effects range from heart rate and blood pressure abnormalities to gastrointestinal distress, while effects on the eyes include tearing, blurred vision, and lens cloudiness with long-term use.

## Carbonic Anhydrase Inhibitors

Carbonic anhydrase inhibitors (oral or drop form; trade names include Trusopt, Diamox, Neptazane) are named after the enzyme carbonic anhydrase, which is found in many tissues of the body, including the eye. Inhibition of its activity in the eye decreases eye fluid production. One of the major side effects of this drug, especially when taken orally (as a pill) can be photosensitivity, which makes the eyes more susceptible to oxidation damage—the last thing someone with glaucoma needs! Other side effects of taking it orally can include kidney stones, numbness or tingling, fatigue, lethargy, loss of appetite, depression, diminished libido, dementia, or nausea. Some people have allergic reactions to carbonic anhydrase.

These drugs are often prescribed with vitamin C, which helps to prevent kidney stones. Anyone with kidney problems should be very cautious in using carbonic anhydrase inhibitors. If you are using oral carbonic anhydrase inhibitors, you should have regular blood testing to make sure your white blood cell counts are normal. The drops tend to have far fewer negative side effects than do the pills. We strongly recommend the drops over the pills.

## Prostaglandin Eye Drops (Xalatan)

Prostaglandin eye drops are a newer treatment that can control eye fluid pressure by increasing outflow of aqueous humor. They have fewer side effects than beta-blocker eye drops. A harmless change of eye color from blue or green to brown may result from use of this medication. Temporarily blurred vision and burning and stinging when drops are instilled are side effects that occur in up to 15 percent of users, but Xalatan is the new drug of choice, espe-

cially for people who don't tolerate the other medications well. These are among the best eye drops
available for treating glaucoma.

## Are the Risks Worth the Benefits?

I hope you're starting to see how the benefits of these
medications may sometimes be outweighed by their
risks and that you'll make sure they're absolutely
necessary before using them. Remember, not all
vision loss in glaucoma is due to high pressure within the eyes.

Aggressive treatment of slightly raised intraocular pressure hasn't had a very good track record of
sight preservation in people with glaucoma. One
research group revealed that although 20 percent of
the adult population has eye pressure above 21 mm
Hg (mercury), only 3 percent of the eyes below 23
mm Hg and only 8.4 percent of those with pressure
above 23 mm Hg have narrowed visual fields.
Attempts to treat glaucoma by lowering eye pressure
are akin to attempts to alleviate heart disease by lowering blood cholesterol. Not only is it not always
effective, but the treatments can prove more dangerous than the disease. An overdose of those potent
medications can cause serious problems.

Most patients don't stick with drug treatment of
glaucoma because of the unpleasant side effects and
the lack of noticeable improvement. In one study,
almost half of patients didn't properly take their
medication or forgot to take them.

## Surgical Treatment of Glaucoma

Surgery is a last-resort treatment for glaucoma, but it may be necessary if there is continuing damage to the optic nerve despite maximum medical therapy. For decades we have seen thousands of patients a year, and based on that experience, we can't recommend strongly enough that you aggressively treat your glaucoma with the lifestyle and nutritional changes outlined in this book before having surgery to treat glaucoma.

You should work closely with your eye doctor in making decisions about glaucoma surgery. He or she will try to determine whether vision loss from glaucoma is likely to affect your quality of life. Your ability to use medications properly will play a role; for example, you may have trouble getting eye drops into your eyes if your hands are shaky, or side effects may be too much to handle. If you have other eye problems, these will also have to be considered.

The surgery done in most cases of glaucoma is called *trabeculectomy*. A pressure-relief valve is surgically created out of the eye's natural tissues. One of the possible side effects of this surgery is that inflammation and scarring can close up the drain following surgery. The most common side effect of glaucoma surgery is bleeding into the eye that usually clears up within a few days.

One study of ninety-three patients with open-angle glaucoma who underwent trabeculectomy showed that about half of the eyes operated on needed more surgery within five years, and that two-thirds needed more surgery within ten years to keep glaucoma under control. Developing cataracts or hastening the development of cataracts is a very common side effect with all eye surgery, but especially with glaucoma surgery.

Two recent studies discovered that a preservative used in glaucoma eye drops, *benzalkonium chloride*, was causing allergic and inflammatory responses in up to half of patients undergoing glaucoma surgery. We'll address this topic at length in Chapter 14, "Basic Eye Care."

A newer surgical procedure that involves implanting a synthetic drain into the eye is showing promise in cases that don't respond to other surgical or drug treatments.

Lasers may also be used to shrink the tissues in the fluid drain to improve drainage, but this is only a short-term solution.

Again, we want to emphasize that the aggressive use of nutritional approaches to glaucoma is especially important, since the medical treatment maze for this disease is complicated and not always effective.

## Nutritional Prescription for Glaucoma

Your best bet for preventing and treating glaucoma nutritionally is to maintain a balanced diet that emphasizes fresh vegetables and fruit, and includes several servings per week of cold-water fish. Eat a variety of low-fat protein, including eggs, turkey, chicken, and soy products such as tofu and tempeh. If you are a vegetarian, be sure you're getting plenty of vitamins A and D and the B vitamins. Avoid rancid oils, hydrogenated oils, and processed meat products such as ham and bologna.

Studies have shown that the blood vessels that feed the retina are not up to par in people who have glaucoma, so one of your primary goals is to improve blood flow to that area. (See Chapter 10 for details on improving circulation.)

Foods to enjoy: blueberries, garlic (to decrease LDL cholesterol), asparagus, eggs, carrots, spinach, cold-water fish, any foods rich in vitamin C, almonds, onions, olive oil (use this in place of other cooking oils), avocados, and watermelon. Keep dietary fat below 30 percent of daily calories. Try to manage the stress in your life so that you stay in balance, get some exercise, and avoid optic nerve toxins like MSG, aspartame, steroid medications, tranquilizer medications, antidepressants (lithium and monoamine oxidase inhibitors), antibiotics, and tobacco.

### Daily Supplements for Glaucoma

Vitamin C: 1,000 mg

Vitamin E: as recommended in your multivitamin

Carotenoids: Use a mixed carotenoid supplement at different times from your ingestion of beta-carotene-rich foods. A mixed carotenoid supplement should contain approximately 25,000 IU of beta-carotene,

1 mg of alpha-carotene, 5 mg of lycopene, 6 mg of lutein, and 0.3 mg of zeaxanthin. (The first detectable sign of optic nerve fiber loss in glaucoma is the dying off of carotenoid pigments from the retina.)

Vitamin A: 5,000–10,000 IU

Quercetin: 1,000–3,000 mg

Rutin: 1,000–3,000 mg (especially helpful if you are using miotics)

Magnesium: 250–400 mg, at bedtime (calcium channel blockers, medications that do the same thing in the body that magnesium does, are used in some cases of glaucoma to open up eye blood vessels. Why use a blunt instrument [the drug] instead of the natural version that works in concert with the systems of the body?)

Vitamin B complex: as recommended in your multivitamin

Vitamin $B_{12}$: 1,000–2,000 mcg (Since it is not well absorbed when taken orally, take it sublingually—under the tongue—or use a nasal spray or gel.)

Zinc: as recommended in your multivitamin

Coenzyme Q10: 90–200 mg (Use with ginger root capsules for added effect if you have low-pressure glaucoma; this will increase your heart's pumping capacity.)

Carnitine: 500 mg, to strengthen the heart's pumping power

Omega-3 oils found in fish. Eat cold-water fish (salmon, mackerel, cod) at least twice a week, or take three to six 1,000 mg capsules of fish oil daily. (DHA, a component of omega-3 oils, is a component of the optic nerve lining.)

Garlic: 1 raw clove with food; or 1,000 mg of the odorless capsules

Coleus (forskolin): 200–400 mg (Coleus is an herbal remedy that has been used for centuries to relax muscles in blood vessel walls, thus easing high blood pressure and ocular hypertension. You can buy capsules under the name *forskohlhii*. It has been shown to significantly decrease eye pressure in drop form, but is not absorbed well and can temporarily cloud vision. If it clouds your vision, stop using it.)

Chromium: 200–600 mg a day if you are using beta-blocker eye drops, to help boost HDL cholesterol

IN SHORT . . .

1. Glaucoma, the "sneak thief of sight," can painlessly progress for some time before it is detected. Damage to the optic nerve causes this disease, and this damage can be due to elevated eye fluid pressure, poor circulation to the optic nerve, or plugging of the fluid drain.

2. While ocular hypertension puts you at greatly increased risk for glaucoma, it does not mean you have it for sure. Aggressive drug treatment of ocular hypertension may do more harm than watchful waiting and tracking of visual field loss, along with nutritional and lifestyle changes.

3. The only symptom of glaucoma is loss of side vision, which can develop into tunnel vision and eventually complete blindness. This painless process often goes unnoticed until there is significant vision loss.

4. A summary of the nutritional "Rx" for glaucoma can be found in Appendix I at the end of this book.

# 6

# Preventing and Healing Cataracts

Cataracts are quite common in aging Americans, affecting two-thirds of those over seventy years of age. Every year Medicare costs for cataract surgeries amount to more than $3.4 billion. As we age, the lenses of our eyes lose flexibility. Because there isn't any cell turnover in the lenses, they have to last a lifetime. By the age of sixty-five, only 40 percent of light rays that hit the eye pass through the lens to the retina. (It's interesting to note that cataracts protect against macular degeneration by blocking light to the retina.) Cataracts are caused by intense sun exposure, poor nutrition, or sugar accumulation in the lens of the eye.

The aspirin-sized lens is held in place by muscles that change its shape when focusing is necessary. In the aging process, the lens becomes unwieldy, inflexible, and thick, and clarity is lost, as is the ability to focus. It feels like looking through a piece of frosted glass, with disturbing glare from bright sun or

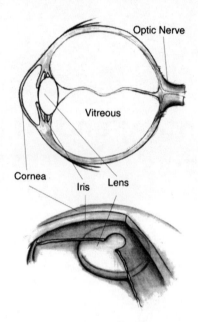

The lens of the eye becomes clouded in people with cataracts.

oncoming headlights. The symptoms are so subtle that many simply think they need new glasses. By the age of eighty, cataract sufferers need a 240-watt bulb to see what they once could with a 60-watt bulb.

As the lens yellows, color vision is altered. Clothes are mismatched or stains go unnoticed by the wearer. Blurred vision can result in falls. Independence may be lost. Family members may mistakenly think the person affected is senile.

Diabetics are prone to cataracts because excess sugar in the blood causes lenses to swell and lose

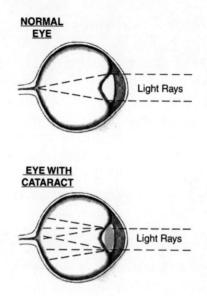

A clouded lens causes light coming into the eye to scatter, creating blurred vision.

transparency. People who live in sunny climates also are more likely to develop cataracts that worsen more quickly than people living in more cloudy areas. Heavy cigarette smokers have cataracts twice as often and at an earlier age than nonsmokers.

Surgical replacement of cataracts is very effective and recovery time is short, but it's always best to use nutritional means and lifestyle modifications to prevent eye problems. Antioxidants, control of blood glucose (in diabetics), and ultraviolet protection with sunglasses and wide-brimmed hats are the best ways to keep the lenses of your eyes clear and flexible.

## Mainstream Treatment for Cataracts

Of all the eye diseases covered in this book, cataracts
are most likely to be surgically treated with excellent
results. As early as the mid-eighteenth century, lenses
clouded by cataracts were removed surgically. The
most cutting-edge technique for the removal of
cataracts is phacoemulsificaton, a procedure that uses
a tiny vacuum tube (called a cannula) inserted into the
lens capsule to ultrasonically fragment the diseased
lens. The fragments are then vacuumed from the eye.
If you take a look at the diagram on page 102, you'll
see the location of the lens. A new lens, called an
intraocular lens, is then inserted into the capsule from
which the original lens was removed.

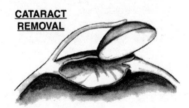

**CATARACT
REMOVAL**

Cataract surgery is a relatively safe, simple surgery in
which the clouded lens is removed and replaced.

Clouded membranes around the lens capsule
may develop during the weeks or months following
cataract surgery. Laser surgery can be used to remedy this problem quickly.

Cataract surgery these days involves so little trauma to the eye that you usually can have both eyes
repaired at the same time.

Correcting blurred vision due to cataracts is an

important preventive measure against falls. Hip fracture is a major risk for older adults with cataracts, who may not see a bump in the pavement or the last step of the staircase. Early-stage cataracts present the greatest risk because a person afflicted with them won't know to be more cautious because vision loss isn't very pronounced.

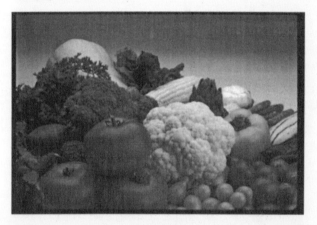

Cataracts cause distorted vision that may become hazy or blurry.

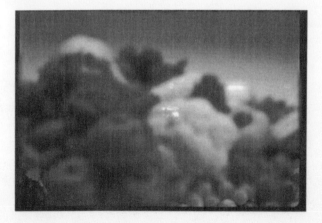

Once you have had surgery, be sure to wear your sunglasses every time you go outdoors. Those who have had lens implants with ultraviolet light filters have more protection. Those who have not had this type of lens implants need to be careful to protect the macula (central retina) from sun exposure. The protection the clouded lens offered is now absent, and the risk of macular degeneration increases dramatically. Needless to say, we strongly recommend you get the lens implants that have ultraviolet light filters.

The bottom line is that you need not live with cataracts or allow them to rob you of your independence. Try the preventive methods outlined in this book for three to six months, and if any of the following symptoms still exist, seek out an experienced eye surgeon:

✓ Vision that is brighter in one eye than in the other (close one eye and check for brightness of view in the other).

✓ Glare in sunlight or dazzling glare from oncoming headlights when driving at night.

✓ Frequent changes in your eyeglass prescription.

✓ A lazy eye that doesn't seem to move as sharply as the other one.

✓ Inability to read, watch television, or participate in recreational activities.

✓ Diminished color vision (difficulty matching socks and clothing, or others telling you your hair is overdyed).

✓ Double vision.

✓ Need to avoid dimly lit areas such as dark restaurants or theaters; need for stronger light bulbs or a flashlight to function at home.

✓ Inability to pass driver's license eye exam.

## Nutritional Prescription for Cataracts

Eat a diet rich in soy, spinach, eggs, asparagus, garlic, and onions. Carrots, cantaloupe, yams, corn, and collard and mustard greens are other foods that will help you keep your lenses clear.

### Daily Supplements for Cataracts

Vitamin E: as recommended in your multivitamin

Vitamin C: 1,000–2,000 mg

Beta-carotene: 10,000–25,000 IU

Vitamin A: 5,000–10,000 IU

Zinc: 15–30 mg (total for the day)

N-acetyl cysteine (NAC): 500 mg, 2–3 times daily between meals

Rutin (a bioflavonoid): 250 mg

Quercetin (another bioflavonoid): 1,000–3,000 mg (This inhibits aldose reductase, which may be a primary cause of diabetic cataracts.)

Chromium: 200 mcg, to help you control blood sugar

Riboflavin: 50 mg (If you need to add to your multivitamin, do so.)

Coenzyme Q10: 30–90 mg

Curcumin (turmeric): liberally as a spice, or taken as a supplement according to directions on the bottle.

IN SHORT . . .

1. Two-thirds of Americans over the age of seventy have cataracts.

2. In cataracts, the flexible, clear lenses become stiff and opaque. It becomes hard to focus, and vision blurs. There is disturbing glare from oncoming head-lights at night and from bright sun. Color vision is altered. In the worst cases, difficulty seeing and recognizing faces can be mistaken for senility and can rob older people of their indepen-dence.

3. Diabetic cataracts are commonly seen. They result from accumulation of excess sugar in the lenses, causing them to swell and become inflexible.

4. Don't hesitate to have cataracts removed. It's a simple procedure that almost always yields good results. As soon as you feel your quality of life is being compromised, talk with your eye doctor about surgery.

5. A summary of the nutritional "Rx" for cataracts can be found in Appendix I at the end of this book.

# 7

# Preventing and Healing Diabetic Eye Disease

Diabetes is much more common than you might think. Eleven million Americans have diabetes, and 40 percent of them show at least mild signs of related eye disease. There are two forms of diabetes: Type I (insulin-dependent), which occurs in children and adolescents; and Type II (non-insulin-dependent), which affects people past middle age.

The juvenile-onset (insulin-dependent) variety is due to destruction of the cells in the pancreas that make insulin. People with this disorder have to monitor their blood sugar levels carefully throughout life and use insulin injections to mimic what their own insulin-producing system would have done: carry sugar molecules into cells to fuel their functions. Without insulin, cells can't get the energy they need. This type of diabetes makes up only a small percentage of diabetics.

In the more common adult-onset variety of diabetes, the body makes insulin, but the cells have

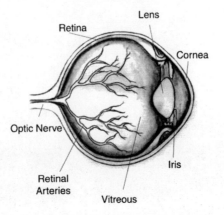

In diabetic eye disease, retinal blood vessels break down, causing damage to the retina itself.

become resistant to it and it doesn't work properly. Not only is there too much sugar in the blood, but there's too much insulin. Adult-onset diabetes tends to occur in people who are overweight and in people with all the symptoms that signal heart disease (high "bad" LDL cholesterol, low "good" HDL cholesterol, and high blood pressure).

Diabetes is a disease with far-reaching implications in the body. Diabetics have more heart disease, kidney disease, blood vessel disease in the extremities, and eye disease than the general population.

Both the lens and the retina are affected by the ineffectiveness of insulin and the excess of glucose in the blood that characterizes diabetes, resulting in macular edema (swelling around the macula), new growth of abnormal retinal blood vessels, and retinal hemorrhage into the vitreous gel that fills up the center of the eye.

The first signs of disease we can distinguish in the eyes of a diabetic are small, berry-like bulges in the capillaries. In later stages, we see small white balls known as "cotton-wool spots" and hemorrhage (leakage of fluid and blood components from capillaries) is visible; the cotton-wool spots are an indication that retinal cells are dying. Chances are, we won't see a patient *just* for these signs because there's no loss of vision yet. This is why it's important for diabetics to have regular eye exams, even if vision seems fine.

If no changes are made in a diabetic's intake of crucial nutrients, the blood vessels to the macula continue to leak, causing surrounding retinal tissues to swell. There may be fatty deposits on the macula, which we can see as yellowish-white streaks. Some blurring of central vision is likely. At this stage, the diagnosis would be *macular edema*.

Left untreated, the disease process leads to damage to the capillaries feeding the retina that is so severe that they become useless, and that part of the eye is unable to get nourishment. In response, the body tries to grow new vessels on the surface of the retina. These weakened vessels can break, leading to hemorrhage into the vitreous humor (the fluid in the center of the eye). Blindness is a very real threat at this point.

Because diabetes is a metabolic disorder that affects every process in the body, the recommendations for reversal of diabetic eye disease start with those proven to help control diabetes. Diabetics have been shown in a number of studies to thrive on exercise and a very low-fat, high–complex carbohydrate diet, or on a low-fat, high-protein, low-carbohydrate diet. You'll have to experiment to find out which one works best for you.

## Mainstream Treatments for Diabetic Retinopathy

As soon as you are diagnosed with diabetes, you should have an eye exam. Be sure the ophthalmologist knows you are diabetic. After that point, you should have yearly eye exams to detect any traces of retinal disease.

To see leaks in retinal blood vessels that can lead to macular edema and destruction of vision cells, the ophthalmologist injects a harmless dye into a vein in the arm. Special photographs are taken of the eye, and the dye clearly shows any leaks. This test is called a fluorescein angiogram.

Two techniques are available to treat different aspects of the disease.

One is laser treatment (photocoagulation), used to seal off leaky blood vessels and control swelling, or macular edema. New blood vessel growth, called retinal neovascularization, is much more delicate than older vessels, and this raises the risk of leaky blood vessels that allow blood to escape into the eye fluid. If your eye doctor finds this is happening, scatter laser treatment can be used to prevent further damage. Loss of sight isn't prevented with laser treatment; it's only delayed for three to four years. Poor dim-light vision and reduced peripheral vision can be side effects of laser surgery. As with any surgical or medical treatment, a careful weighing of risks and benefits is necessary. No mainstream treatment is totally without risk.

The second technique that your eye doctor may use if he or she finds that you have had a hemorrhage into the vitreous humor that fills the middle of the eyeballs is called a vitrectomy. Precision instruments are used to remove the blood from the vitreous jelly.

Aspirin may be recommended to increase retinal blood flow, but we recommend you avoid it. A large-scale study of 3,711 diabetics showed no advantage for those who used aspirin over those who didn't. As we mentioned previously, aspirin can aggravate existing eye problems by causing leaky blood vessels, and it can be very harmful to the stomach.

## Nutritional Prescription for Diabetic Eye Disease

Treatment for any complication of diabetes begins with good control of blood sugar levels through diet, supplements, stress management, and exercise. The Ten Steps to Restoring Vision and Vitality outlined in the first chapter are your foundation for controlling diabetes. The majority of adults with Type II diabetes can stay off insulin and diabetes drugs if they're willing to change their lifestyle.

This means regular exercise (at least thirty minutes five times a week and preferably more) and a willingness to virtually eliminate sugar and refined grains from the diet. Refined grains include white and whole-wheat bread (look for whole-grain bread), cakes, cookies, chips, pasta, and white rice. We strongly recommend that you not substitute aspartame (NutraSweet) for sugar. It's a known eye toxin, and a dangerous chemical with too many side effects for anyone struggling to stay healthy and save vision. If you have a craving for sweets, try some fresh fruit.

The mainstay of a healthy diet for stable blood sugar is vegetables, with protein (eggs, meat, fish, fowl, tofu) and complex carbohydrates (brown rice, whole grains) as an accompaniment.

In view of the side effects of diabetes drug treatments, insulin problems, and poorly controlled blood sugar—including heart disease, kidney disease, and vision loss— it seems well worth it to make sacrifices to maintain good health.

Until new lifestyle habits are established and you're in a routine, blood sugar should be monitored at least four times a day. It's important to notice what raises or lowers your blood sugar and to keep track of these factors. High blood pressure also should be monitored and well controlled to keep blood vessels healthy. Nearly all high blood pressure can be lowered through diet, exercise, supplements, and stress management. Everything we recommended above for treating Type II diabetes will help lower your blood pressure as a beneficial side effect.

We ask our diabetic patients to keep a detailed

daily journal for at least three months, recording their blood sugar, blood pressure, everything they've had to eat or drink, amount of exercise, as well as what has happened during the day. This is a powerful and illuminating exercise in self-awareness on every level, and we highly recommend it for anyone with chronic health or emotional problems.

Eat plenty of bioflavonoid-rich foods, like blueberries, cherries, raspberries, and red onions.

## Daily Supplements for Diabetic Eye Disease

Some of the supplements listed here, as well as the recommended dietary guidelines above, will improve insulin sensitivity and lower blood sugar levels, so it's very important to monitor blood sugar when you start this supplement program and make the necessary adjustments.

Vitamin C: 2,000 mg (This may alter the color of urine strips; work with a health care professional if you are diabetic and think you need more than 2,000 mg of vitamin C daily.)

B vitamins: as recommended in your multivitamin

Vitamin E: as recommended in your multivitamin

Beta-carotene: as recommended in your multivitamin

Quercetin: 500–1,000 mg

Chromium: 100–200 mcg, to help balance blood sugar

Vanadyl sulfate: 10–20 mg, to help stabilize blood sugar

Magnesium: 400 mg, at bedtime, to help control blood pressure

N-acetyl cysteine: 500 mg, 2–3 times between meals

Omega-3 oils from cold-water fish twice a week

Garlic: 1 raw clove, with food, or 1,000 mg of the odorless capsules

Zinc: as recommended in your multivitamin

Carnitine: 500 mg

Alpha lipoic acid: 500 mg in divided doses (Studies are confirming that this powerful antioxidant reduces diabetic symptoms such as nerve damage and dangerously high blood sugar due to insulin resistance. It also protects the lenses from formation of diabetic cataracts. Remember to monitor your blood sugar closely because it can cause a significant drop in blood sugar.)

IN SHORT . . .

1.  Type II (adult-onset) diabetes is a very common disease in aging Americans and usually strikes those who are overweight and have high blood pressure, high "bad" LDL, and low "good" HDL cholesterol levels. The body still makes some insulin, but it doesn't do its job of carrying glucose into cells for energy. Levels of insulin and blood sugar can be dangerously high.

2.  Type I diabetes involves destruction of the cells of the pancreas that make insulin. Injections of insulin need to be timed appropriately throughout the day so that glucose can enter the cells and fuel their function.

3.  Diabetics are more prone to cataracts and blindness due to new blood vessel growth or hemorrhage over the retina than the general population. It's crucial that you see your eye doctor as soon as you are diagnosed as diabetic and to go for thorough checkups every year.

4.  Eating a low-fat, high-fiber diet, avoiding sugar and refined carbohydrates, losing excess pounds, exercising, and learning to cope with stress can keep diabetes under control without drugs.

5.  It helps to keep a journal of what you're
    eating, how you feel, and blood sugar
    levels for the first few months after
    you're diagnosed. Frequent monitoring
    and close control of blood sugar can
    help to stave off eye problems.

6.  Laser treatments can preserve sight in
    those with leaky eye vessels. Vitrectomy
    is used to "clean up" hemorrhages into
    the vitreous humor that fills the eyeball.
    Aspirin may do more harm than good
    for those with diabetic eye disease.
    Your best bet, as always, is to use diet,
    exercise, and supplements to control
    your diabetes.

7.  A summary of the nutritional "Rx" for
    diabetic eye disease can be found in
    Appendix I at the end of this book.

# 8

# Preventing and Healing Retinitis Pigmentosa

Retinitis pigmentosa (RP) includes fourteen types of disorders involving the pigmented cells of the retinal surface (*epithelium*). These visual pigments are part of the cells of the retina and are responsible for the eye's sensitivity to light. They are shed and replaced by new pigment cells. People with retinitis pigmentosa have abnormal pigment cells that clump together on the retina and can't be flushed out of the eye. Only a fraction of people with eye diseases suffer from RP, and the fact that it is so rare has impeded the progress of working towards a cure.

Symptoms begin with night blindness, often starting in childhood. A progressive loss of side vision occurs in the person's third decade of life. Tunnel vision (by the age of forty or fifty) and eventual total blindness are the end result of retinitis pigmentosa. It's a difficult disease to have because there is no known mainstream medical treatment. The work being done on retinal cell transplantation is

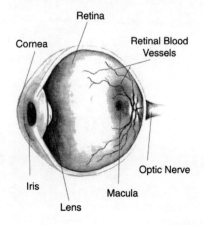

Retina
Cornea
Retinal Blood
Vessels
Optic Nerve
Iris
Macula
Lens

Retinitis pigmentosa is a rare eye disease that affects the pigmented cells in the retina of the eye.

promising, but we still don't know whether it will provide us with a cure for RP. Up to half of RP cases are genetically linked.

Half of those with RP will develop cataracts, and most have problems focusing, reading, and adjusting to bright light. Headaches are also common, as are the anxiety, anger, and depression that result from the knowledge that vision will fade and eventually disappear.

If you have been diagnosed with RP, you should know that you are not helpless. You can slow the progress of the disease substantially by using the advice in this book. Researchers are looking into theories that an inflammatory process that affects many systems of the body is what causes the damage done by RP. It may be an autoimmune disease like arthritis, where the body develops antibodies (its natural disease-fighting agents) against its own tissues, doing them harm as it would a dangerous bacterial or viral invader.

The most important thing RP patients can do while we seek causes and cures is to give the eye all the tools it needs for maximum antioxidant protection. Look at Chapter 3 for advice on how to boost glutathione levels. You also should carefully read and follow our guidelines in Chapter 9 on digestive tract problems. Supplementation of digestive enzymes (bromelain is particularly gentle and effective) as well as *Lactobacillus acidophilus* and *Lactobacillus bifidus* bacteria can make a big difference for those who suffer from gas, bloating, or other symptoms of irritable bowel (diarrhea, constipation, intestinal cramping). Those symptoms mean you aren't efficiently absorbing the nutrients from the food you eat.

One-third to one-half of those with RP have a family history of the disease. Here are some of the predisposing factors for retinitis pigmentosa in those without a genetic history:

✓ Photosensitizing drugs (including Mellaril, thiazide tranquilizers, tetracycline, sulfa drugs, and diuretics)

✓ Intense sunlight (ultraviolet and blue-violet sun rays bleach night vision chemicals, reducing night vision)

✓ Diets high in unsaturated oils (such as those from corn and safflower)

✓ Diets high in hydrogenated oils (found in chips, cookies, and margarine, for example)

✓ Diets low in the essential fatty acids found in fish and fresh vegetables (Omega-3 and omega-6 fats are necessary for renewal of night vision cells.)

✓ High or low thyroid

✓ Liver or pancreatic disease

While there are no known cures for retinitis pigmentosa, there are many steps those with this disease can take to save their sight. As with any other eye disease, the foundation for better eye health is in our Ten Steps to Restoring Vision and Vitality, found in the first chapter. Get those in place first and then add in the special supplements and therapies we suggest in this chapter for the well-being of your eyes.

## Mainstream Treatments for Retinitis Pigmentosa

Unfortunatly, there are no surgeries or drugs to reverse this disease. Cataracts often occur in people with RP, and these can be removed. Scatter laser treatments are sometimes used to bring down swelling of the macula or to seal off new blood vessels that impede vision; this is not a permanent solution, however.

Some exciting work is being done with hyperbaric oxygen treatments, where the RP patient inhales pressurized oxygen. Several studies have shown that hyperbaric oxygen slows the progression of the disease. You can ask your eye doctor about this, but remember that it's still in its experimental stages, and unfortunately it's very expensive.

Prescription magnifiers and low-vision aids, as described in Chapter 15, are helpful in making the most of your visual abilities.

Early detection is important so that those with RP can immediately begin eating foods and using supplements known to slow its progression. See Chapter 11 on prescription drugs and eye disease for details on drugs that cause photosensitivity. These drugs should be avoided. Further research is needed to discover whether these drugs actually cause cases of RP that are not genetic.

## Lifestyle Prescription for Retinitis Pigmentosa

✓ Eat plenty of garlic, onions, asparagus, and eggs and supplement vitamins E and C along with alpha lipoic acid and N-acetyl cysteine to raise your glutathione levels.

✓ Eat lutein-rich foods like spinach, kale, collards, and mustard greens. A lutein/zeaxanthin supplement derived from marigold petals is a good idea.

✓ Avoid unsaturated oils.

✓ Incorporate at least twenty minutes of brisk walking into each day's schedule.

✓ Use stress-reduction techniques to lower elevated levels of adrenal hormones, which can weaken eye capillary walls and lead to swelling and tissue damage.

✓ Alternate consumption of lutein-rich foods with beta-carotene-rich foods. For example: For breakfast, have half a cantaloupe with your oatmeal; at lunch, have a salad of spinach, onions, and tomatoes. Eat small amounts of fat and zinc with your beta-carotene to enhance absorption.

✓ Have cold-water fish such as cod, salmon, or sardines two or three times a week. Walnuts are another good source of omega-3 fatty acids.

✓ Wear wraparound sunglasses to protect your eyes from ultraviolet rays.

✓ Avoid tobacco. Don't smoke and don't be around people who smoke.

✓ Avoid alcohol because you need to keep your liver as healthy as possible so it can make plenty of glutathione and supply the eyes with vitamin A.

✓ Avoid drugs that stress the liver, which is almost all prescription drugs. One of the most commonly used over-the-counter drugs that stresses the liver is acetaminophen (Tylenol).

✓ Avoid vitamins containing iron.

✓ Avoid photosensitizing drugs (see Chapter 11).

✓ Avoid refined sugars and refined carbohydrates.

✓ Avoid eye toxins such as monosodium glutamate (MSG) and aspartame (NutraSweet).

✓ Avoid chronic stress; get professional help if you need to.

### Daily Supplements for Retinitis Pigmentosa

Vitamin E: as recommended in your multivitamin

Vitamin C and bioflavonoids: 1,000–2,000 mg and 250–400 mg, respectively

Beta-carotene: as recommended in your multivitamin

(Take all of the above antioxidants together, so they can re-energize one another as they work.)

Lutein/zeaxanthin: 6–12 mg, at different times from ingestion of beta-carotene

Zinc: as recommended in your multivitamin

B vitamins: as recommended in your multivitamin

N-acetyl cysteine (NAC): 500 mg, 2–3 times between meals

Quercetin (another bioflavonoid): 500–1,500 mg (This inhibits aldose reductase, a cause of cataracts; RP commonly leads to cataracts.)

Bilberry, grapeseed, and cranberry extracts: (These are other good sources of bioflavonoids, which help vitamin C to strengthen capillaries in the eyes.) Follow directions on the container

Coenzyme Q10: 30–200 mg

Magnesium: 300–400 mg, to reduce calcium deposits on the retinas and improve circulation

L-Carnitine: 300–1,500 mg

Cayenne pepper capsules: (These provide a potent stimulant, dilate blood vessels, increase circulation, improve cholesterol ratios, and decrease blood clotting.) Take 1–2 capsules with meals.

Ginkgo biloba: 120–360 mg, to improve circulation

Alpha lipoic acid: 100–300 mg, to keep glutathione levels high

Taurine: 1,000 mg (taken with 800 IU vitamin E, divided into 2 doses) if you have the autosomal dominant form of RP, or if you have Usher's syndrome.

If you have digestive problems, try supplemental digestive enzymes to maximize absorption of essential fatty acids and vitamin A. We'll address digestive enzymes in detail in Chapter 9 on digestion.

Those who know early they have RP should start right away with a diet and supplement program to maximize the benefits, even if vision loss hasn't started.

---

   IN SHORT . . .

1. Retinitis pigmentosa is actually a number of different disorders, all of which result in clumping of retinal proteins, loss of side vision, tunnel vision, and eventual blindness. The first symptom is usually night blindness starting in childhood or early adulthood.

2. Although there is currently no cure, those with RP can take control through nutritional and lifestyle changes and use of supplements. The progression of the disease can be slowed significantly with these interventions.

3. A summary of the nutritional "Rx" for retinitis pigmentosa can be found in Appendix I at the end of this book.

# 9

# There Is No Good Nutrition without Good Digestion

Ingrid has been coming to us for eye care since we started our practice here in Los Angeles. Her eyes have always been sharp, and only since she turned sixty-seven last year has she needed glasses for reading. Vitamin supplementation and good food choices have been part of her life for at least ten years, and the benefits are obvious. She's tall, strong, and vibrant.

At her checkup Ingrid says she's not feeling as well as usual. Her stomach has been upset, and antacids haven't helped at all. She often suffers from gas, constipation, and bloating. After meals she has been feeling as if there's food stuck deep down in her throat. I note in her chart that her retinas don't look as good as they normally do, and ask Ingrid if she's been sticking to her regular routine of exercise, diet, sunglasses, and supplements. "Of course," she replies. "Why? Is something the matter?"

I explain that her retinas are looking a little lack-luster and that if everything besides her digestive health is the same, she might consider using some supplements to improve digestion. I caution her against the use of antacids and acid blockers such as Tagamet and Zantac. "Too much acid isn't your problem. As you age, your stomach produces less and less acid," I tell her. "That can affect whether the nutrients that come into your body get absorbed. A lack of stomach acid can cause nutritional deficiencies."

I send her home with some suggestions: probiotics like *Lactobacillus acidophilus* to keep her large intestine populated with friendly bacteria, and digestive enzymes to help break down food in her small intestine.

I run into Ingrid at the local health food market about six weeks later. She practically sprints across the produce aisles, her shopping basket overflowing with leafy green stuff. "Those supplements work wonders. I feel so much better and my digestive problems are gone." I'm continually amazed and gratified at how some basic awareness of the body and a few simple, natural steps can create profoundly positive changes in our health.

## The Perils of Poor Digestion

Why a chapter about digestion in a book on eye disease? Well, by now I think you're beginning to understand how intimately everything is related in your body. If your digestion is poor, you can be eating all the right foods and taking all the right supplements and still not get any of those precious nutrients to your cells.

As you pass your fiftieth birthday, you're likely to be producing significantly less stomach acid than you did at age twenty-five. According to some estimates, between 24 and 37 percent of adults aged sixty to eighty suffer from lack of digestive acid (also known as *atrophic gastritis*), but our guess is that it's much higher. We have found that the majority of our patients over fifty benefit greatly from some hydrochloric acid (HCl) with meals. The acid produced in your stomach is a key player in the thorough breakdown of food. Those who don't have enough stomach acid often can't digest fiber-rich whole foods or vitamin pills, and turn to highly processed foods to meet their energy needs. Vitamin and mineral deficiencies often already exist because of a history of poor food choices, and poor digestion compounds the problem.

When you can't completely digest your food, your body can't absorb the vitamins it contains. Vitamins are locked into foods, and your body's digestive system uses hydrochloric acid and enzymes as keys that release them and allow them to be absorbed into the bloodstream. Stomach acid is also responsible for the activation of enzymes needed for digestion as food travels into the small intestine and colon. In older people lowered levels of vitamins $B_2$, $B_6$, and $B_{12}$, as well as decreased absorption of zinc from vegetable sources, may be in large part due to low stomach acid. Undigested food travels farther along the digestive tract than it's meant to, and gas and bloating can result.

## Enzymes: The Raw and the Cooked

When you take a bite of a mixed meal (containing protein, carbohydrate, and fat), perhaps a turkey burger on a whole grain bun with lettuce, tomato, onion, and avocado slices, digestion begins in your mouth. An enzyme secreted by your salivary glands called *salivary amylase* starts breaking down the carbohydrates in the food. Your tongue and teeth work together to mix food with saliva. The grinding and crushing actions of your teeth also prepare food for absorption through the membranes of the small intestine. In addition to the enzymes your body makes to break food down into usable parts, fresh whole foods themselves contain enzymes that help your body to digest them. Cooking at above 118 degrees Fahrenheit wet heat, as in boiling, or 150 degrees Fahrenheit dry heat, as in baking, denatures or kills enzymes. They are defunct, unable to do their work. You can see right away that if you eat nothing but cooked food, you won't ever get the help of the enzymes contained in raw foods.

Enzymes are proteins that are integral to nearly every biochemical process in the body. In order for them to be active, they need plenty of vitamins and minerals, which act as *coenzymes*, important parts of enzyme machinery. Some minerals are part of enzyme complexes, and if there is a deficiency, then a shortage of that enzyme can result. (Yet another good reason to eat well and take your supplements!) Over five thousand enzymes are known to exist in living creatures. They have a variety of functions, including metabolism, elimination of toxins, and digestion.

It's said by some experts that if your body has to do all the work of enzyme-making, without help from those present in food, it eventually will become exhausted, and enzyme production will fall. Without proper amounts of enzymes, some of the food you eat can remain undigested and cause you problems such as food allergy (if large food particles leak into the circulation) or formation of too much gas in the large intestine (caused by friendly bacteria gorging on undigested food).

Let's get back to your mouth. It's happily chewing the bite it just took. Thorough chewing is important to good digestion. Not only does it break food down mechanically and enzymatically; it also sends a message to the salivary glands, stomach, liver, and pancreas to get started with their secretions. Take your time at meals and take small bites. If you tend to have problems with intestinal gas, eat slowly and chew each bite fully so you'll swallow less air with your food.

Many older people have tooth and gum problems that make it hard to chew fresh, raw foods. Living on tapioca pudding isn't the answer. If you use a blender and a juicer in food preparation, you can enjoy fresh fruit and vegetable juices, and you can puree cooked beans and vegetables to make nourishing soups.

Modern juicers allow you to include the fiber-rich pulp in the juice.

Supplemental coenzyme Q10 can help improve the health of painful gum tissue. If you do have to cook your vegetables or make soups to ease chewing, be sure to supplement with digestive enzymes (see page 143).

## The Real Reason for Heartburn

The esophagus has smooth muscle in its walls that contracts to help transport your bite of food to the stomach. Whatever enzyme activity has been preserved works towards partial digestion of the food in the upper part of the stomach. Food's natural enzyme activity gives the stomach a break, loosening some of the bonds that must be broken before nutrients can be accessed by the body.

Hydrochloric acid and a protein-digesting enzyme precursor (*pepsinogen*) are released from specialized cells in the stomach lining into the stomach. Pepsinogen is transformed to pepsin, the protein-digesting enzyme, when exposed to stomach acid. Hormones are also released into the stomach at this point. They respond to what foods you have eaten and regulate accordingly how fast the stomach empties into the small intestine. Digestion of fats takes much longer, so a fatty meal will stay in your belly for quite a while. Protein takes a little less time, and carbohydrates are digested most quickly. Secretion of other enzymes farther along the digestive tract also is dictated by these hormones.

Stomach acid is highly concentrated, designed to break down food so that enzymes can act on it efficiently in the small intestine. Even before food hits your stomach, the smell and taste of it sets your salivary glands and acid-producing glands to work. Stomach acid is essential for efficient digestion, and yet it gets unfairly blamed for causing heartburn, ulcer, and other kinds of gastrointestinal upset.

More than half of people over forty have heartburn at least once a month. Heartburn occurs when food mixed with acid leaks up into your esophagus, causing feelings of a lump in the throat, chest pain, or burning in the stomach. Recently, acid-reducing medications like Zantac, Tagamet, and Pepcid became available over-the-counter for relief of heartburn. Antacids like Tums, Rolaids, and Mylanta have been the traditional pharmacological remedies for heartburn, also called *gastroesophageal reflux*. These drugs block stomach acid, and I believe they contribute to malnutrition in older people. They are the last thing most people need for heartburn.

Contrary to what the companies that make these drugs would like you to believe, it's the rare case of heartburn that's caused by overproduction of stomach acid. In many cases, it's a *lack* of stomach acid that's to blame. As you get older and your stomach acid production falls, food sits in your stomach for longer and longer periods during the digestion process, increasing the chance of it being burped back up. Your esophagus doesn't have a thick mucous lining to protect it like the stomach does, so even the smallest bit of acid causes burning.

A weakened sphincter muscle between the stomach and the esophagus can also contribute to discomfort. Drugs (including calcium channel blockers prescribed for heart pain, nicotine, and beta-blockers often prescribed for high blood pressure) can cause this muscle to relax when it shouldn't. High levels of stress, obesity, and old age can have the same effect. Over time, repeated bouts of heartburn can loosen the sphincter muscle permanently.

How can you prevent heartburn? Here are some pointers:

✓ Follow the Ten Steps presented in Chapter 1, and avoid fried foods or excessive amounts of fatty foods. Fat in the stomach sends out hormonal messengers that cause the stomach to empty more slowly.

✓ Don't eat a lot at a sitting. Snacks are actually a good idea. It's best not to be famished when you sit down to eat.

✓ Lose excess weight.

✓ Don't eat on the run or right before or after exercise. If you're stressed, blood flow and energy are being shunted away from the gastrointestinal system. This can decrease acid production. Make mealtimes into little oases of peace in your day.

✓ Drink alcohol in moderation, never more than two drinks a day.

✓ Here's a tough one: Cut way down on chocolate, which can be very aggravating to some heart-burn sufferers.

✓ Don't lie down right after a meal.

✓ Work towards reducing the number of prescription and over-the-counter drugs you are taking.

✓ Reduce stress by exercising or taking classes in meditation, yoga, qi gong, or Tai Chi. A hot bath also can help you control a "stomach-clutching" response to stress.

## Natural Remedies for Heartburn

If you do have an attack of heartburn, try natural remedies before reaching for antacids. A glass of room-temperature water; the juice of raw cabbage or potato; aloe vera; herbal teas such as fenugreek, slippery elm, comfrey, licorice, and meadowsweet (no lemon, lukewarm); fresh papaya; or fresh banana are all recommended by Earl Mindell, R.Ph., Ph.D., a well-known expert on natural alternatives to prescription drugs.

The last thing you need is antacid tablets or acid-blocking pills. You may experience temporary relief, but your stomach is likely to produce another surge of acid an hour later so that you have to take more antacids. Antacids are not the harmless drugs the advertisements would have you believe they are.

They cause acid rebound, they block the absorption of nutrients, they interact with several prescription drugs (including some antibiotics, aspirin, and the heart drugs Cardioquin and Quinalan), they slow digestion, and they can cause diarrhea or constipation. People who take a lot of antacids tend to have more urinary tract infections.

The myth that Tums are a good source of calcium is not only irresponsible but dangerous to women who think they're boosting their calcium levels and preventing osteoporosis. Antacids actually block calcium absorption, so at best the calcium in them is supplementing what is depleted by the antacid.

## The Real Cause of Stomach Ulcers

Your stomach has a thick mucous lining to protect it from acid; when a bacterial infection known as *H. pylori* (short for *Helicobacter pylori*) erodes this lining and exposes the stomach wall to the acid environment inside it, stomach ulcer results. Low stomach acid may make the stomach more susceptible to an *H. pylori* infection.

No matter how low your acid secretion is, it is powerful enough to burn a hole in exposed stomach lining. The fact that stomach ulcers are caused by bacteria rather than overproduction of stomach acid is a fairly new discovery. It's no coincidence that $H_2$ blockers (another name for stomach acid-blocking drugs such as Tagamet, Zantac, and Pepcid) went over-the-counter as heartburn medicines at about the same time this discovery was made: these drugs were originally prescribed for treatment of ulcers.

*H. pylori* bacteria are found in 70 to 80 percent of cases of stomach ulcer, and 90 percent of cases of duodenal ulcer. (The duodenum is the first part of your small intestine, just outside the stomach.) In 50 percent of people who suffer not from ulcer but from heartburn, stomach distress, or indigestion, *H. pylori* is the cause. If you have indigestion, ask your doctor to test you for an *H. pylori* infection. If you do have this bacteria in your gastrointestinal tract, it needs to be eradicated before you can enjoy good digestion. A course of antibiotics (usually tetracycline and amoxicillin) and a bismuth preparation (such as Pepto-Bismol) should do the trick.

If you want to try a natural remedy for banishing *H. pylori*, Dr. Earl Mindell recommends deglycyrrhizinated licorice lozenges (chewable) between meals, and odorless garlic capsules with meals for at least three weeks and as many as six weeks.

If you're one of those people who suffer regularly from heartburn and the remedies we've suggested here don't work, be sure to get a checkup from your doctor. Sometimes heartburn can be a symptom of undiagnosed heart disease.

## Increasing Stomach Acid

You have many choices when it comes to enhancing your stomach acid safely and naturally:

✓ Eat a balanced diet of unprocessed, organic whole foods. Try to have a green salad with raw vegetables once a day, so you can reap the benefits of live enzymes that are disabled by cooking and processing.

✓ Chew your food thoroughly.

✓ Drink a glass of lukewarm water thirty minutes before meals. Very hot or cold liquids interfere with secretion of acids and enzymes. You may want to try mixing a tablespoon of apple cider vinegar in with a cup of the premeal water. Vinegar is acidic, making it a good digestive aid.

✓ Try tinctures of bitters like goldenseal or gentian. Mix in a one-to-seven ratio with water.

✓ Try a stomach acid supplement sold in health food stores called betaine hydrochloride (HCl). Some brands also contain pepsin for better protein digestion. Try a 250–300 mg tablet with food, and gradually increase the dose to two or three tablets a meal. If your stomach burns, you've taken too much. Be sure to take it *with* a meal.

## The Small Intestine, Pancreas, and Liver

Let's continue along the digestive tract. Once partly digested food (*chyme*) has been churned around in your stomach for about thirty minutes, it moves in small amounts through another sphincter that leads to your small intestine. Most of the work of digestion and absorption of food is done in the ten-foot-long small intestine. The pancreas and liver secrete enzymes into the first section of the small intestine (the *duodenum*) that are crucial for good digestion. These enzymes include more amylase for digestion of starches, protease for protein breakdown, and lipase for fat digestion. They also neutralize the acid in the chyme as it passes so it won't harm the rest of your digestive tract. Aging people make enzymes less effectively, and those who have depended on antacids for years are likely to make even fewer enzymes than predicted for their age. If you have gas and bloating after meals, it can't hurt to try a digestive enzyme supplement with amylase, protease, and lipase. Some also include enzymes for digestion of lactose (milk sugar) and cellulose (the insoluble fiber in plant foods that can cause flatulence after eating beans).

The liver is truly an amazing organ. It's the largest gland in the body. It makes and stores its own natural antioxidants like glutathione, coenzyme Q10, and superoxide dismutase. It metabolizes proteins, carbohydrates, and fat; it neutralizes toxins and drugs; and it produces a half-liter of bile a day, which is stored in the gallbladder for secretion into the duodenum when food comes through. Bile is 97 percent water and contains bile salts made from cholesterol. These salts work on fats in the chyme, breaking it into small particles that are easily digested by lipase (a fat-digesting enzyme). The bile salts then are recy-

cled back to the liver to be used again. Without
enough bile, fat digestion is poor and the absorption
of fat-soluble vitamins such as A, E, and D is limited.

Taking too many prescription or over-the-counter
drugs can hurt your liver over the long run.
Acetaminophen (Tylenol, for example) is one of the
worst offenders. Alcohol, fatty foods, and exposure
to chemical toxins like gasoline and pesticides can
stress your liver and make it less able to perform all
its functions, including the manufacture of bile.
Under ideal circumstances, the liver can clear blood
of toxins without any problem. If it's overloaded with
drugs, alcohol, unhealthy foods, environmental toxins, or any combination of these, it can't keep up.
The overflow of toxins is allowed to leak into the circulation to wreak havoc elsewhere.

Gallstones are a fairly common occurrence in
Americans. Blockage of the flow of bile by these
stonelike deposits can cause fat and fat-soluble vitamins to pass through the system undigested.
Gallstones are created when there's too much cholesterol and not enough *lecithin*, another component
of bile. The typical American diet that's low in fiber
and high in fat and sugar is to blame. Supplemental
lecithin can be bought at your health food store to
help insure you against gallstones. It's also used as a
natural cholesterol-lowering agent.

Keeping your liver healthy and happy is an
important part of good health. Following the Ten
Steps in Chapter 1 will help keep your liver healthy.

If you know your liver is going to be stressed, you
can use the herb milk thistle. Its active ingredient,

silymarin, directly supports the liver by protecting cell membranes from breakdown, and helps in the formation of new liver cells and production of bile. The bioflavonoid catechin, vitamin C, alpha lipoic acid, and N-acetyl cysteine (a precursor to glutathione) are other substances you can use in supplement form to keep your liver healthy.

## Leaky Gut Syndrome and Food Allergy

The chyme that once was a turkey burger continues along, now mixed with pancreatic enzymes and bile that busily work to break down large molecules into small ones. Contractions of the muscular walls of the small intestine pump chyme along. In a healthy gut, the protein, carbohydrate, and fat molecules that are the end result of digestion seep through the intestinal walls to the liver, and then into the circulation. Transport systems for these molecules through the membranes that line the inside of the small intestine are varied and complex, designed to let out only what the body can use and to retain all else for eventual excretion in the feces.

If your nutrition is poor or you have taken antibiotics, the gut membranes can become more permeable than they should be. Large molecules not meant to travel in the bloodstream escape through "leaks" in the gut. Food allergies are the result of the body's immune response to these molecules, which it sees as hostile invaders. Over time, the food allergies cause more irritation to the gut, creating a vicious cycle of inflammatory reactions throughout the body and chronic digestive problems.

Food allergies generally go undiagnosed in mainstream medicine, but we have seen a world of problems clear up when people eliminate offending foods from their diet. Strictly speaking, these types of reactions to food are "sensitivities," not allergies in the sense that hives or hay fever are, but for the sake of simplicity we use the generic term of allergy to describe the problem.

Gordon is a good example of someone with undiagnosed food allergies. He hasn't been feeling well lately and says that it's been literally years since he really felt good. "I have to lie down for an hour at the office after lunch," he confides. "My head feels fuzzy after I eat. And the cramps I get in my guts are excruciating."

"What does your doctor say?"

"Not much. I go in there with a list of complaints as long as my arm. Rashes, hemorrhoids, gas, you name it. They've run thousands of dollars' worth of tests and found nothing. I'm taking Tagamet and antacids, but they help only for a little while. I guess I've pretty much resigned myself to being like this for the rest of my life."

It sounds to me as though Gordon has some food allergies. I ask him to try eliminating wheat and dairy products, the two most common offenders, to see if he feels better. "What'll I eat?" he asks in a panic. "I can't give up pizza!"

I persuade him to try it for two weeks. He reluctantly agrees, but in that time his skin clears, and his gas and bloating disappear. When he eats wheat again, his symptoms don't return, but when he drinks a glass of milk for the first time in two weeks, he has terrible stomach cramps, bloating, and gas, an indication that he has a sensitivity to milk, and probably dairy products in general. Gordon feels that giving up dairy products is a small price to pay for relief of his symptoms.

How do you know if you have a food allergy? It isn't easy to tell because food allergy symptoms can crop up in any system of the body. Many patients we talk to who later discover they have a food allergy are always feeling a little "off" with nasal allergies, asthma symptoms, rashes, a general feeling of depression or exhaustion, and gastrointestinal complaints, and they have been frustrated by doctors who can't find any specific ailment.

Although wheat and dairy products are the most common culprits, others include citrus fruit, nightshade family plants (tomatoes, potatoes, eggplant), and food additives, preservatives, and dyes. Some children seem to be particularly sensitive to dairy products and food dyes.

If you think you might have food allergies, try an elimination diet. This involves systematically eliminating the foods you eat daily or almost daily for ten to fourteen days, then adding them back into your diet one at a time. Keep a diary of how you feel throughout. Once you've gone without an allergenic food for a few days, the allergic response to it will be much more pronounced when you reintroduce it.

It's interesting to note that the foods you're allergic to are usually the ones you crave. That's because your body's response to the allergen can make you feel a little "high." Your adrenals kick out hormones that raise your pulse and make you more alert as your body prepares to defend itself against the unwelcome invader. Those with food allergy usually can name a food (or two or three) they absolutely couldn't do without, which are the most likely to be those you're allergic to.

If you do have an allergy to your favorite food, don't despair. You don't have to give it up completely. After you have avoided it for a few months, you may be able to enjoy it once or twice a week without ill effects. As soon as you go back to daily consumption, though, symptoms are likely to recur.

Lack of stomach acid and digestive enzymes, bacterial infections, systemic yeast infections (*candidiasis*), chemotherapy, trauma, or excessive stress all can contribute to leaky gut syndrome. If you're interested in learning more about food allergy, refer to the excellent book *Optimal Wellness*, by Ralph Golan, M.D. His chapter on this topic goes into great depth and is a wonderful resource.

Following my supplement recommendations and eating well will do a lot for a leaky gut.

## Colon Health, Friendly Bacteria, and Yeast

If all goes well along the length of the small intestine, the majority of digested matter left to enter the large intestine or colon is waste and water. Bile pigments and insoluble fiber are concentrated, as excess water is reabsorbed into the body through the walls of the large intestine. Propelled by muscular contractions, feces move to the descending colon, where they give the body the signal that it's time to eliminate.

Constipation is epidemic among those who eat the typical American high-fat, low-nutrition diet. Following our Ten Steps in Chapter 1 carefully should spare you the discomfort of hard, difficult-to-pass bowel movements.

Did you know that there are four hundred different microorganisms residing in your small intestine and colon? These friendly bacteria (also called *flora*), including *Lactobacillus acidophilus* and *Lactobacillus bifidus*, feed on carbohydrates that come into your gut. Fruits, vegetables, grains, and milk sugar (lactose) are their daily fare. In return for room and board, friendly bacteria fight unfriendly bacteria. Breakdown of carbohydrates by friendly bacteria produces lactic acid and other substances that make the intestinal environment unpleasant for harmful organisms. Intestinal flora are also important sources of B vitamins and vitamin K.

The bacteria *Candida albicans*, or yeast, also resides in the healthy gastrointestinal tract. It is harmless when there are plenty of good bacteria around to keep it under control. This is the same yeast that causes vaginal yeast infections. If balance isn't achieved, yeast can become overgrown and cause problems throughout the body.

One of the most common ways to get a yeast overgrowth is to take antibiotics. Antibiotic medications kill off friendly bacteria along with whatever bacteria was causing the illness. Without the resistance of your friendly bacteria, or probiotics, yeast can become overgrown. Steroid medications and other drugs that suppress the immune system also allow yeast to thrive. Sucrose, or refined sugar, is yeast's favorite food, and those who eat a lot of it are at risk for intestinal yeast infection. If you aren't making enough digestive enzymes or stomach acid, it's more likely that undigested food will reach the lower small intestine and colon, giving yeast more nourishment to grow and multiply.

How can you tell if you have yeast overgrowth? As in food allergy, which affects many systems of the body at once, there are often multiple symptoms and a feeling of general unwellness. If you must take antibiotics or steroids, or if you have frequent vaginal yeast infections, you can try supplementing your intestinal flora to keep yeast overgrowth at bay.

## Probiotics for Intestinal Health

Whether or not you have a yeast problem, irritable bowel symptoms such as intermittent constipation and diarrhea with bloating and gas may indicate a shortage of friendly bacteria. Avoid antibiotics unless absolutely necessary. Eating foods rich in fiber and snacking on yogurt containing live bacteria (and no added sugar) should boost populations of lactobacilli. You also can use probiotic supplements, sold as acidophilus or probiotics in the refrigerator at your health food store. These might include *Lactobacillus acidophilus, Lactobacillus bulgaricus,* and *Bifidobacterium bifidum*. You need to refrigerate them whether they are liquid or in capsules. Take them according to the directions on the bottle.

IN SHORT . . .

1. If you have problems with heartburn or slow digestion, you may not be making enough stomach acid.

2. To aid digestion, eat whole foods and chew well.

3. To enhance stomach acidity, drink a glass of lukewarm water thirty minutes before meals. Add a tablespoon of apple cider vinegar to the water if needed.

4. To enhance stomach acidity, try supplements such as tinctures of gentian or goldenseal, 1 part to 7 parts water, or betaine hydrochloride tablets (HCl), starting with 300 mg with meals and increasing as needed.

5. Don't overeat or eat "on the run."

6. Manage chronic stress.

7. Enzymes produced in your salivary glands, stomach, pancreas, and small intestine are important players in digestion. If you tend to have indigestion often you can try supplementing with amylase, protease, and lipase at meals. If it's beans or vegetables that cause you problems, try cellulase, which is sold commonly as Beano; if milk upsets your gut, you can use lactase, sold under the brand name of Lactaid. Other brands should be available at your health food store, and you may find an

enzyme supplement that contains all of these enzymes.

8. *H. pylori* infection is a common cause of heartburn, indigestion, and stomach ulcer. Your doctor can easily see if you have this bacteria in your system and can cure it with antibiotics and a bismuth preparation such as Pepto-Bismol. If you want to avoid antibiotics, try garlic and licorice.

9. The liver secretes bile to break down fats for energy. This breaking-down also frees up essential fat-soluble vitamins. Drugs and other toxins can overwhelm the liver to the point where it can't do a good job. Milk thistle is an effective liver-supporting herb.

10. Food allergy is a common consequence of leaky gut syndrome. Try an elimination diet if you suspect you suffer from food allergy.

11. Your colon plays host to four hundred different strains of friendly bacteria. These probiotics perform important functions and should be maintained. Lack of friendly bacteria can lead to yeast overgrowth in the intestines. Avoid antibiotics whenever possible and eat unsweetened "live" yogurt. Supplements containing probiotics can be used as well, and should always be used for the two weeks following a course of antibiotics.

# 10

# Keeping Your Blood Vessels Strong

Now that you know how important good digestion and absorption of nutrients is to healthy eyes, let's take a look at your nutrient delivery system, otherwise known as your circulatory system. The cells of your eyes are fed with oxygen and nutrients through tiny blood vessels; if these are clogged or damaged, guess what? Your eyes literally start to die. That's how important good circulation is to clear vision, and why we're going to take you on an extended journey through the circulatory system. But first let's introduce you to Fred.

Fred came to us for a checkup because for a few months he had noticed that his eyeglasses weren't strong enough, and he was concerned because he had been in for a new prescription just a year ago. Fred is a go-getter, an overachiever who has had great success in his professional life. He's one of those energetic people who thrive on the kind of stress the rest of us would rather avoid. He loves to eat, he smokes a pack of cigarettes a day, and has a couple of martinis when he gets home from the office. He's always felt fine and been healthy, so he has never worried about his health.

But when Fred walked into the office on the day of his appointment, we hardly recognized him. He had gained a few pounds, and he looked sallow and exhausted. Still, he managed an enthusiastic greeting. As I examined him, I asked him how things were going.

"Not great," he said. "My vision is getting foggy. I look at things that should be straight, and they're bent. I went for my physical two months ago, and they prescribed three different drugs because I have high blood pressure and high cholesterol. They flipped out when I told them I had some chest pains. I guess now that I'm over fifty, everything is catching up with me."

"How do the drugs make you feel?" I asked.

"Awful. I'm tired all the time, and for the first time in my life I'm impotent. I can't tell you how bad that feels, Doc. It makes me feel old, like it's all downhill from here." He started to cough. "Oh, and they want me to quit smoking and switch from martinis to red wine. I'm not a red-wine kind of guy. And they want me to exercise, but who has the time?"

After the exam was finished, I had to tell Fred that he had the first signs of macular degeneration, a disease of gradually failing vision. I explained that I could see from the condition of the blood vessels in his eyes that his circulation wasn't great. The age spots on his retinas showed that left alone, his eyes would most likely continue to deteriorate, with loss of central vision a distinct possibility. Fred was shocked. "What can I do, Doc? I'll do anything. I can't lose my sight."

I told Fred that if he was going to save his vision, he needed to make changes in lifestyle even more drastic than his internist had asked for, and that I needed 100 percent cooperation. Fred said he would give 200 percent if it would save his vision, and made an appointment with our staff nutritionist. She created an individually tailored program of diet, supplements, and exercise for healing his eyes. We also asked him to work with his internist to get off the prescription drugs as his health improved because we knew they would only aggravate his eye problems.

Six months later, Fred returned to see us, and this time he looked like his younger, healthier self. He had lost his sizable belly. His skin was smooth, and his color was wonderful. Best of all, he was smiling.

"Dr. Rose!" he hollered when he saw me. "You saved my life! I'm off all the drugs. My blood pressure and my cholesterol are perfect. I kicked the cigarette habit and cut my work hours. I'm playing racquetball with a friend from the office and," he whispered conspiratorially, "I'm not impotent anymore."

"That's great, Fred," I replied, "but how are your eyes?"

"Oh, right, they're fine, they're great. My vision isn't bent anymore, and my old glasses are working fine again." When I checked Fred's eyes I could see very little sign of the circulation problems that had shown up earlier, and told him that as long as he stuck with his new lifestyle, his eyes would be fine. There are millions of people afflicted with the same problems as Fred. High blood pressure and blood cholesterol, heart pains known as angina, and clogged blood vessels throughout the body are epidemic in America. And yet, if you take care of your circulatory system, you can avoid these problems almost entirely.

Once you understand the miraculous nature of the system of blood vessels that your body uses to bring oxygen and nutrients to all its cells, we hope you'll want to do everything you can to keep it healthy. We don't want you to change your lifestyle out of fear of becoming sick; do it because you want to enjoy as many happy, active years as possible. It can be a positive, life-enhancing choice.

## Let's Take a Journey through Your Bloodstream

Blood brings life to your cells. It's a unique fluid that carries vital substances throughout the body to every cell. Blood carries

- Oxygen.
- Nutrients such as vitamins, minerals, and amino acids.
- Immune cells such as white blood cells for defense against infection.
- Substances that cause blood to clot when there is an injury.

- Substances such as cholesterol for repairing injuries to blood vessel walls.
- Dozens of hormones that regulate bodily functions.
- Waste products your cells produce, such as carbon dioxide and urea.

Ninety-one percent of your blood is water, which is one very good reason why we want you to drink plenty of clean water every day, and why that is one of the Ten Steps described in Chapter 1. All told, blood makes up 8 percent of your body weight.

Arteries carry oxygen-laden blood from the heart to the rest of the organs, while the veins bring it back once its oxygen has been unloaded. Every twenty-six seconds, our arteries and veins recirculate about 5.25 quarts of blood from the heart and lungs to the organs and tissues and back again.

## The Arteries: Your Nutrient and Oxygen Delivery System

We'll start our journey through the bloodstream in the left side of the heart. This half of the heart muscle is divided from the other half by a thick wall called the septum. Although the two halves of the heart beat in synchrony, they function as separate pumps, so we'll look at them separately.

The blood within the atrium, the top chamber of the left side of the heart, is bright red, indicating that it is saturated with oxygen. As it contracts, the blood rushes through a valve into the ventricle, the lower half of the left heart. The sound of this valve closing is the familiar "lub" of the heart sound. The ventricle contracts almost immediately after the atrium does, and when another valve closes behind the blood, the "dub" heart sound is heard.

Each heartbeat pumps about a third of a cup out into your arteries. The big artery we've passed into, the aorta, is just the beginning of a huge system of arteries running throughout the body. Arteries have muscle in their walls that contract to help rush blood along to where it's needed. The aorta branches out into smaller arteries. A healthy artery is much more than a channel for blood to flow through. There are several layers, all of which play their own roles in the vessel's health and disease.

## Not Just a Simple Tube

The arteries aren't just simple tubes that blood courses through. They have three layers, each with its own function and its own type of cellular structure.

The inner wall (endothelium) of the artery is a smooth membrane packed with special receptors for substances needed to feed and repair itself and the tissue behind it. As molecules such as cholesterol (for cell-building) and growth factors (to control cell growth) whiz by in the blood, endothelium receptors identify and "catch" them, bringing them through to the central layer of the artery. Some cells that make up the endothelium secrete substances that can cause the artery wall to constrict or expand, while other substances affect the clotting of blood.

The middle layer of the artery is made of tough connective tissue and smooth muscle that moves blood along in a wave-like motion. This is the location of the lumps and clumps called *plaques* and *lesions*, that block the arteries. The smooth muscle of this inner layer contracts when you are excited, stressed, or angry, and relaxes when you are relaxed. This is why stress and anger can contribute so significantly to a heart attack.

The outermost layer of the arteries is rich in blood vessels, and brings nutrients and oxygen to the other layers of the artery. Just as the heart muscle needs its own blood vessels because it can't absorb what it needs from the blood that pumps through it, the blood flowing through the arteries is "off-limits" to the artery wall. These structures have their own separate blood flow.

## Exchanging Oxygen and Nutrients for Waste

As vessels continue to branch off the large arteries, they become smaller in circumference. These smaller vessels are called arterioles. Branching from these are even smaller vessels called capillaries.

Capillaries number in the billions, and they are responsible for letting what each cell needs out of the bloodstream. Simultaneously, wastes from that area of tissue that surrounds the capillary enter the blood so that they can be excreted. The density of capillaries in your muscle is 2,000–3,000 per sq. mm!

A capillary is only the thickness of a human hair, and the membrane that lines it is only one cell thick. Red blood cells pass through in single file. Healthy capillary membranes are porous enough to let nutrients and oxygen in and wastes out, but not so much that vital blood components and proteins can escape the bloodstream.

## Back to the Heart

Now the blood, having given up most of its oxygen and nutrient supply, and loaded with waste products including carbon dioxide, travels out of the capillaries and into small veins, called venules, for the journey back to the heart.

The venules converge into the veins. There is no muscle in the walls of the veins; blood pools in these vessels, and the blood pressure is much lower than in the arterial system. Blood is drawn back to the heart by a pressure gradient, in a kind of suction similar to what happens when you drink liquid through a straw. You create negative pressure with your mouth, which draws fluid up the tube against gravity. The muscles of your arms and legs help to actively pump blood back towards the heart. This is why exercise, or even body movement of any kind, is so important to good circulation. Your blood will circulate back to the heart even if you aren't moving your body, but it certainly moves better when *you* move.

## From the Right Heart to the Lungs

Loaded with wastes and low in oxygen, the blood returns to the right side of the heart. *Lub!*—through the right atrium; *Dub!*—through the right ventricle, and on into the lungs, where the vessels again branch out into minuscule capillaries so that oxygen can pass into the blood and carbon dioxide can pass into the lungs. The carbon dioxide is exhaled. Newly oxygen-laden blood travels from the lungs through what is called the *pulmonary* (meaning "lung-related") vein and back into the left heart, where our journey began.

## Lost on the Circulatory Highway

Sarah is in her late sixties, a widow, and very independent. Her great love is painting seascapes near her home in Santa Monica. "Dr. Rose," she said, "no matter which way I look, there's a dark tunnel around what I see. I can still see, but I'm afraid it will get worse and I'll have to give up my painting."

I asked Sarah if her health was generally good. "Except for a touch of high blood pressure, yes," she said. "My doctor gives me pills, and I hardly notice a difference except that I have to get up two or three times at night to use the bathroom. Still, the doctor says I have to lose fifty pounds before I can go off the medication. I just don't think I'll ever get there. He says I should exercise too, but I'm not sure how to start. It's been so long."

"What about your diet?" I asked.

"Oh, I've been so good about it. I eat almost no fat at all. Just pasta and bread. All those low-fat foods, like cheeses and skimmed milk and saltine crackers. They make some nice no-fat desserts that I just adore, thank goodness! I know I should eat more veggies and fruit. I do like to have a muffin at breakfast with a pat of butter." Sarah thought she was doing the right thing for her health by avoiding fat, but fat would have been almost preferable to her diet of refined white flour and sugar.

As I examined Sarah I saw the telltale signs of circulatory glaucoma: constricted blood vessels behind her retinas, low fluid pressure, and a pale optic nerve. I knew that the drugs she was taking were diuretics, and the frequent urination they caused was the reason her blood pressure had normalized. It hadn't helped her eye vessels, and had probably made her problems worse. When you flush too much fluid from the system, vital electrolytes and water-soluble vitamins are flushed out as well.

Nor were her blood vessels well nourished by her diet of white flour and sugar, so it was a double whammy. I knew that if she took steps to improve her nutrition, Sarah's vessels would repair themselves and her vision would improve.

During Sarah's follow-up visit, after she had been on a program of diet and exercise for three months, her vision had stopped deteriorating. Within six months her eye vessels looked stronger and better able to carry blood to her optic nerve. After nine months she brought us one of her paintings, a gorgeous view of the California sunset. "Thanks to you, I won't miss any of these," she said.

# What Can Go Wrong with Arteries

You can imagine that if the big, strong arteries coming out of the heart are narrowing due to an accumulation of plaques and lesions, other blood vessels are equally affected, and your billions of capillaries will start dying off.

Here are some of the many ways that blood vessel blockage can affect you:

- When the blood vessels to the brain are blocked, the result is a stroke or loss of mental function.

- Loss of blood to the legs causes painful cramps with very little activity.

- Loss of blood to the fingers and toes causes numbness and tingling, and in some diabetics may even result in amputation.

- Loss of circulation to the blood vessels that feed the eyes can result in macular degeneration and other eye diseases.

- Loss of circulation to the liver doesn't allow it to cleanse your blood of toxins the way it should. If your blood circulates back through the heart still loaded with waste matter, it will contribute to damaged blood vessels.

- Blockage of the carotid arteries in the neck, which bring blood to the head, can cause strokes and loss of sight.

If arteries are clogged, the capillaries don't get the blood flow they need to stay healthy, and they become leaky. Circulation is impeded, and cells die from lack of oxygen and nutrients. Tiny and delicate, capillaries are vulnerable to becoming clogged by clots that come loose from artery walls (this is called *thrombosis*) or to becoming encrusted with unhealthy calcium deposits. All of these problems prevent the capillary from doing its work.

If the capillary membranes become too fragile due to lack of sufficient oxygen and nutrients, red blood cells leak through and cause hemorrhage, and fluid leaks through and causes swelling. This is one way that poor circulation to the delicate vessels that nourish your eyes can lead to macular degeneration and other eye diseases.

## Putting Risk Factors into Perspective

There are a number of well-known "risk factors" for artery disease. High blood cholesterol, high blood pressure, obesity, and family history of heart disease are probably most familiar to you. But some of these risk factors have been given more importance than they deserve because research and publicity about them has been driven by drug company funding, advertising, and education programs. That's right. Those screening programs at your local clinic or drugstore are sponsored by your friendly drug company, whose main mission is to get you to take their drug.

The research studies showing that high cholesterol and high blood pressure must be lowered to treat heart disease is funded by drug companies. If these risk factors were that important on their own, we would have eradicated heart disease a long time ago because cholesterol-lowering and hypertension drugs handle those symptoms very effectively. There must be more to it.

Let's take a more unbiased look at heart disease risk factors and put it in some perspective.

High blood cholesterol is an indication that you have heart disease, but it is an *effect* of heart disease, not a cause. The real culprit is *oxidized* LDL ("bad") cholesterol and a component of some cholesterol called lipoprotein(a), identified by Linus Pauling and Mathias Rath, M.D., as an important factor in clogging blood vessels. When low antioxidant levels allow oxidation damage to arteries, lipoprotein(a), which has a sticky quality, comes along and tries to repair the damage. This is good news if you're about to spring a leak in an artery, but bad news if you're low on antioxidants and the lipoprotein(a) just keeps piling on. If your arteries aren't damaged, normal cholesterol floating through your blood is not going to hurt you.

Let's look at what actually happens in the artery when it becomes oxidized or clogged:

- The vessel wall is injured.
- The blood rushing through the injured vessel sends blood cells called platelets to the site of the injury, forming a kind of clot. This is the body's normal healing response.

- Due to the same factors that injured the artery, the injury doesn't heal quickly, and the small clot attracts more platelets and secretes a substance that causes the vessel to constrict. This is an attempt to control blood flow past the injury, but it can also result in further injury to the vessel. If you're under a lot of stress, and have a lot of adrenaline coursing through your body, your blood is more likely to clot too much around an injury.

- Other substances at the injury site cause tissue growth and cell migration into the injury, which are healthy responses in a normal body. But if the blood is overly thick, there is too much buildup of tissue growth at the site. White blood cells also stick to the area and accumulate cholesterol from the bloodstream. This cholesterol-filled cell is called a macrophage.

- All of the cells conglomerated around the initial injury continue to produce growth factors, causing tissue to grow. Fibrous connective tissue develops to support it.

- A fully developed lesion contains a cholesterol core. The rate at which lesions develop varies a great deal, so that some might become life-threatening in a year while others might be harmless for decades.

- When a lesion is large enough to limit blood flow to crucial organs, these symptoms begin:

  - heart pain with activity, known as angina

  - problems with memory or movement

- visual blackouts

- the shooting pains of blocked blood vessels to the legs (intermittent claudication)

- Stress on a lesion (as can happen with constriction of the artery or turbulent blood flow) can tear or rupture a lesion. Pieces of the plaque are set loose in the bloodstream, where they can become lodged in other vessels. This is often the cause of a heart attack or stroke.

## How to Reduce Injury to Blood Vessels

Diseases of the blood vessels are largely caused by normal healing mechanisms gone awry. There's a lot of exciting research going on that is showing us what truly reflects a person's risk of blood vessel disease. We're learning about the importance of antioxidants, homocysteine levels, fibrinogen levels, glutathione levels, and magnesium in determining your risk of cardiovascular disease. Understanding what puts you at risk will give you the tools to stay free of disease.

### Antioxidants

The first event in the chain that leads to clogged blood vessels is some sort of injury to the smooth inner wall of the artery, the endothelium. This can be caused by many kinds of toxins, but the biggest culprits are cigarette smoking, exposure to pesticides and air pollutants, and rancid (oxidized) fats and hydrogenated oils. What is common to all of these is that they are major players in the production of free radicals. Antioxidant nutrients buffer harmful free radicals before they can damage your arteries. Lack of these vital nutrients, including vitamins C, E, beta-carotene, the bioflavonoids, selenium, and precursors to the body's supply of glutathione, allows free-radical damage to run rampant in your body. After dozens of excellent studies, it's clear that low levels of antioxidants significantly raise your risk of blood vessel disease.

## Homocysteine

Homocysteine is an amino acid that is formed when your body metabolizes or processes methionine (an amino acid that's part of protein foods). Homocysteine is toxic, and normally a healthy body breaks it down before it can build up. To keep homocysteine levels low, you need B vitamins, especially vitamin $B_{12}$ and folic acid. Homocysteine levels rise when you're nutritionally deficient and don't get enough B vitamins, or enough choline and betaine, important factors that help B vitamins perform their functions. More than twenty studies on two thousand subjects have shown that homocysteine levels are higher than normal in people with heart disease.

## Magnesium

Magnesium is a mineral that is plentiful in unprocessed, whole foods like grains, legumes, and colorful vegetables. Most of us don't get anywhere near enough of it in our diets. A U.S. Department of Agriculture study showed that only 25 percent of 37,785 people were meeting the Recommended Dietary Allowance (RDA) for magnesium (which is minimal to begin with). In one study, people suffering from high blood pressure or decreased strength of the heart, both signs of coronary artery clogging, were given intravenous magnesium, which lowered their blood pressure and reversed their heart muscle dysfunction. Magnesium helps to keep blood flowing smoothly, elevates HDL ("good" cholesterol) levels, helps maintain blood pressure, and regulates heartbeat. It helps keep your bloodstream free of harmful calcium that can deposit in artery lesions by promoting the absorption and metabolism of calcium. Magnesium works in opposition to the constricting effects of calcium throughout the body, helping to keep blood vessels relaxed and open. We all could use more magnesium, and if your diet includes processed foods, you're not getting enough.

## Fibrinogen

Fibrinogen is a component of your blood. It plays a role in clotting, which on the outside is the formation of a scab over a cut, for example. If there is too much fibrinogen in your blood, it becomes too sticky and can contribute to stopped-up blood vessels as well as build onto existing plaques along the arteries. If the oil in your car gets too thick and gummy, your car doesn't run as well, and the blood in your body is no different. Fibrinogen, which like cholesterol is a vital substance, becomes harmful when you are under excessive stress, if you smoke, or if you are obese. Obviously, weight loss and quitting smoking are important steps to take to keep your arteries healthy, and stress reduction is a goal all of us strive towards.

To lower your fibrinogen levels, try eating more cold-water fish, olive oil, garlic, and foods rich in fiber, especially whole grains. Some studies show promising effects of moderate amounts of alcohol, particularly red wine.

## Glutathione

Glutathione is an antioxidant produced mainly in the liver, to the tune of about 14 g per day (about $3\frac{1}{2}$ tsp.). It works synergistically with vitamin C and vitamin E. People who are healthy as they age have high levels of glutathione. In people suffering from heart disease, diabetes, and arthritis, the concentration of glutathione in the blood is low.

This most basic antioxidant neutralizes free radicals and other toxins, stabilizes red blood cells, and improves the function of the immune system. Glutathione is one of the best-known promoters of eye health. Low glutathione levels are associated with nearly every type of eye disease. Since it is an unstable molecule that hasn't successfully been stabilized for supplement use, the best way to raise your glutathione levels is through a good diet and the supplement N-acetyl cysteine, which is a building block of glutathione.

## Lysine and Proline

The amino acids lysine and proline provide protection, along with vitamins C and E, to artery walls by removing accumulations of lipoprotein(a). According to the work of Linus Pauling and Mathias Rath, the lysine and proline make the normally sticky lipoprotein(a) smooth, so it can slip off the blood vessel wall.

# Roadblocks to Healthy Blood Vessels

Instead of worrying so much about eliminating all fat and cholesterol from your diet, try to eliminate oils that easily become oxidized. Stick with stable vegetable oils like olive and canola. In small amounts saturated fats are not at all harmful. Coconut oil is certainly not the villain it's been portrayed as by the vegetable oil industry, and it's wonderful for baking. A little butter is also fine. Both coconut oil and butter are vastly preferable to the hydrogenated oils found everywhere in processed foods, which are just plain toxic to your blood vessels. The point is to keep your overall fat consumption moderate, or low if you have existing blood vessel disease, and avoid the unsaturated and hydrogenated oils.

If you want healthy blood vessels, please stay away from that sugar bowl. In fact we suggest you put flowers in the sugar bowl. Put down that white-flour roll, that bagel, and ditch the white-flour spaghetti. Refined sugar, also called sucrose, and white flour (even the enriched kind) are both sources of calories without vitamins and minerals. Your body has to use its precious stores of nutrients to process these empty foods. Think of them as "anti-nutrients." If you fill your belly with white flour and sugar, there's less room for healthy, nutrient-dense foods, and you will be deficient in the nutrients essential to blood vessel health.

Did you know that the number of cases of artery disease in a population is correlated more to sugar consumption than to fat or cholesterol consumption? A possible mechanism is in the depletion of crucial nutrients and the artery clogging that results. We don't want you to become extreme about this. Sugar is OK in moderation. But that means a couple of times a week, not a couple of times a day.

## Stress

When your body is subjected to chronic stress, the chemicals your body releases under stress become toxins, especially to your blood vessels. This is why we strongly recommend meditation, which reduces stress and helps us learn to keep our emotions balanced.

## Excess Estrogen

Excessive estrogen, or estrogen not balanced by progesterone, can increase a woman's risk of strokes caused by blood clots. It is also known to cause and aggravate eye problems, probably due to small clots in the blood vessels and capillaries of the eye, and has a tendency to cause edema, or water retention.

## Nutritional Prescription for Clear, Strong Blood Vessels

Limit your consumption of white sugar, refined flour, and "bad" oils that are unstable and easily oxidized. Keep fat and oil intake moderate.

Increase your intake of fiber-rich foods, especially whole grains and fresh vegetables. Increase your intake of glutathione-boosting foods: cold-water fish, eggs, asparagus, garlic, onion, and soy foods.

### Daily Supplements for Clear, Strong Blood Vessels

Vitamin C: as recommended in your multivitamin, and up to 10,000 mg (10 g) if needed

Vitamin E: as recommended in your multivitamin

Magnesium: as recommended in your multivitamin

Folic acid: as recommended in your multivitamin

Vitamin $B_6$: as recommended in your multivitamin

Vitamin $B_3$ (niacin) in the form of inositol hexanicotinate: 100 mg

Vitamin $B_{12}$: 1,000–2,000 mcg, sublingually or intranasally

N-acetyl-cysteine (NAC): 500 mg, 2–3 times

Lysine: 300–500 mg, 3 times

Proline: 300–500 mg, 3 times

CoQ10: 30–90 mg

Carnitine: 100–150 mg

Betaine hydrochloride: a 250–300 mg tablet, increasing the amount if needed, with meals, to improve digestion and absorption of B vitamins

---

 **IN SHORT . . .**

1. Without a healthy circulatory system, the rest of your body can't enjoy good health.
2. Avoid pesticides, cigarettes, rancid oils, and sugar.
3. Antioxidant supplementation is crucial for keeping your circulatory system healthy.
4. Low levels of glutathione and other antioxidants, and high levels of homocysteine and fibrinogen, allow the body's healing responses to get out of hand, creating blood-stopping clumps and lumps in the arteries.
5. Magnesium is essential to healthy blood vessels.
6. A summary of the nutritional "Rx" for healthy blood vessels can be found in Appendix I at the end of this book.

# 11

## Are Your Prescription Drugs Making You Go Blind?

There are times when you need to use prescription drugs. In many instances they save lives and help people who are in great pain to get on with their lives without undue suffering. The other side of the coin is that we have become a culture that expects a miracle pill for every illness. Even the illnesses that can be avoided by lifestyle adjustments, that we ourselves are able to control without the aid of prescription drugs, are most commonly treated with powerful medications rather than good advice. Because drugs work so quickly and alleviate uncomfortable symptoms (usually without addressing the underlying problems), it seems we literally can have our cake and eat it, too. So why not live it up, eat whatever we like, neglect exercise, and pop some pills when our blood pressure rises and our blood cholesterol levels shoot through the roof?

If you've gotten this far along in this book, you already know that prescription drugs can have very harmful effects on your body's delicately balanced systems. Many commonly used prescription drugs can negatively affect nutrient levels, circulation, essential fatty acid balance, fluid balance, and kidney and liver function. The very powerful properties that make these substances work are what cause all this mayhem in your body.

Most of the doctors who prescribe prescription drugs are trained to pluck a group of symptoms out of context, knowing next to nothing about how the patient eats or sleeps, whether he or she is in an abusive relationship or has money problems. When we talk to our patients about the medications they take every day, many of them know nothing about how the drugs work or what negative effects they can have. More often than not they don't even know what the drugs they swallow daily are called, referring to them as "heart pills" or "cholesterol pills." This is an indication that we have become too comfortable with this system, living the lifestyles that make us ill and expecting nothing less than magic pills to alleviate our suffering.

This is not to say that medical doctors are not a knowledgeable group of professionals or a tremendously valuable resource. The point is that you need to be informed about what you are putting into your body. Take an active role in your own health care, questioning your physician, probing and digging for information. At the very least, read the package inserts in any drugs you take and ask the pharmacist to help you understand it thoroughly.

Doctors are inconvenienced by patients who do this. Managed care has drastically cut the amount of time doctors can spend with patients simply talking and answering questions. Remember that the health care system is there for you and that you have every right to get as much support as you need.

In John Robbins' excellent book on health care, *Reclaiming Our Health,* he describes a study from Yale University run by Bernie Siegel, M.D. Patients who survive cancer, Dr. Siegel remarks, are those who shun the traditional role of passive patient. There was "a 100 percent correlation between the head nurse's opinion of the patient and the long-term survival rates." The patients who made the most trouble were those whose outcomes were the best!

## Look Out for Your Own Interests

Pharmaceutical companies are billion-dollar industries focusing on the bottom line of profit. If a drug is potentially lucrative, testing for safety and efficacy can be cursory at best. Prozac, an antidepressant prescribed to millions of Americans, is a good example. Most patients on this drug take it for at least a few months, but 86 percent of the patients involved in the clinical trials of the drug were treated for three months or less. Not much was learned about Prozac's long-term effects before it was approved. Now, with millions on the drug, it is becoming apparent that Prozac can permanently damage the systems it was designed to regulate and that severe rebound effects once the drug is stopped are not uncommon.

Natural plant-derived substances such as vitamins and minerals cannot be patented, so they are not as profitable to manufacture and distribute as synthetic drugs. There is no incentive to research and develop safe, gentle natural medicines when the highly potent synthetic versions can be exclusively distributed for decades at high prices.

Have you ever leafed through a medical journal? The pages are dotted with glossy, full-page ads for the latest prescription drugs. Representatives from drug companies visit hospitals and doctors' offices to peddle their wares to physicians, handing them free samples for their patients. Drug companies pay leading researchers huge sums of money for studies crafted to prove their latest creations work; they provide honorariums for continuing medical education lectures and contract physicians as "consultants" for huge salaries.

The only way for you to get out of this loop is to be well informed and to take charge of your own health. Avoid taking prescription drugs whenever you can, choosing instead to use gentler remedies such as changes in diet, herbs, supplements, and other natural therapies. If you *need* to use antibiotics to cure a serious infection or if you *need* a short course of nonsteroidal anti-inflammatory drugs to get through a bad spell of arthritis pain, or if you *need* to have chemotherapy for cancer, do so. Know all there is to know about potential side effects and drug interactions and get back to a drug-free life as quickly as you can. (But never stop a medication you've been taking without consulting with your doctor.)

In the rest of this chapter we're going to talk specifically about which prescription drugs can cause or worsen eye problems, and can result in loss of vision.

## Know Your Medicines

Prescription drugs are known by their generic name and their brand name. For example, Advil is the brand name for ibuprofen and acetaminophen is the generic name for Tylenol. Once the patent expires on a drug, other companies have the right to manufacture and sell it under its generic name or other brand names. Some of the other brand names for ibuprofen or drug combinations that include ibuprofen are Motrin, Genpril, Haltran, Midol, and Nuprin. In the information we give you will be the generic name and one of the more common brand names.

It's important to know both the generic and brand name of any drug you use. Look at the bottles to find out what the substance is called, or ask your doctor or pharmacist to give it to you. If you can't remember them or pronounce them, write them on a slip of paper you keep in your wallet or purse. In any medical emergency it's important for those who care for you to know what drugs are in your system, so that dangerous drug interactions can be avoided.

## Drugs That Negatively Affect Nutrients

You already know that good nutrition is the most important step you can take for healthy eyes. Problems can arise when you take prescription drugs that affect the absorption or transport of these vital nutrients. Whether by disrupting fluid balance, flushing needed minerals from the body (both characteristic of diuretic blood pressure medication), or carrying fat-soluble vitamins out of the body unabsorbed (as do the drugs used to lower high blood cholesterol), these drugs rob your eyes of needed vitamins and minerals and can affect vision adversely.

## Drugs to Lower Blood Pressure

Diuretics are very commonly prescribed to lower blood pressure, which they do by decreasing the fluid volume in the blood vessels and making you urinate more frequently. One of the negative effects of diuretics is that minerals are lost with all that urination, and minerals are essential to good circulation and thus to good eye health. With some diuretics, retention of calcium in the body is increased, while too much magnesium is lost in the urine. Calcium is a vasoconstrictor (it causes blood vessels to constrict), and if it isn't properly balanced with the vasodilating mineral magnesium, circulation can be impeded. That means trouble for your eyes.

Here are the names of some of the diuretics used to lower blood pressure:

## Thiazide Diuretics

chlorothiazide (Diuril, Diurigen)

hydrochlorothiazide (Esidrix, HydroDIURIL, Hydro-Paroretic, Ezide)

bendroflumethiazide (Naturetin, Clothiazide, Aquatensen, Enduron)

benthiazide (Exna)

indapamide (Lozol)

hydroflumethazide (Diucardin, Saluron)

trichlormethiazide (Metahydrin, Naqua, Diurese)

polythiazide (Renese)

quinethiazone (Hydromox)

metolazone (Zaroxolyn, Mykrox)

chlorthalidone (Thalitine, Hydroton)

## Loop Diuretics

furosemide (Lasix)

bumetanide (Bumex)

ethacrynic acid (Edecrin, Edecrin Sodium; prescribed for lowering of intraocular pressure in glaucoma)

torsemide (Demadex)

## Cholesterol-Lowering Drugs

These types of drugs bind cholesterol and remove it from the circulation to be excreted in the feces. Fat-soluble vitamins that are transported on cholesterol molecules are swept through unabsorbed. These drugs are known as statins. Some examples of statins include Lovastatin (Mevacor), Clofibrate (Atromid), and Gemfibrozil (Lopid).

## Drugs That Can Interfere with Nutrient Absorption

These are drugs that can cause damage to the lining of the stomach and intestines, which may interfere with nutrient absorption, or that interfere with digestion in such a way as to block absorption of nutrients:

antibiotics (Erythromycin, amphotericin B)

nonsteroidal anti-inflammatory drugs (NSAIDs)

$H_2$ blockers (Tagamet, Pepcid, Zantac)

antacids (Tums, Mylanta)

## Photosensitizing Drugs

There are dozens of prescription drugs that make the skin and eyes more sensitive to sunlight. If you must use these medications, take special care to protect your eyes and your skin from sun exposure. Oxidation reactions that occur when sunlight strikes the eye play a significant role in the development of cataracts and macular degeneration, and photosensitizing drugs compound these reactions. There are some researchers who believe that these drugs may cause retinitis pigmentosa in some people. Always check your drug information insert (if you aren't given one, ask for it) to find out if it can cause photosensitization. If you have eye problems or are at risk for them, do everything you can to avoid these drugs:

thiazide diuretics

loop diuretics

potassium-sparing diuretics

carbonic anhydrase inhibitors (used to treat glaucoma)

antiarrhythmic drugs used to regulate heartbeat in those at risk for heart rhythm problems (flecainide, digoxin, quinidine, procainamide, lidocaine, amiodarone, and verapamil, for example)

blood-thinning drugs such as heparin (Warfarin)

nifedipine (Procardia)

antihistamines (cyproheptadine, diphenhydramine)

NSAIDs (phenylbutazone, ketoprofen, naproxen)

anti-infectives (most antibiotics and sulfa drugs)

auspinone (anti-anxiety drug)

venlafaxine, netazodone (antidepressants)

fluvoxamine, paroxetine, sertraline (antidepressants/anti-anxiety drugs)

zolpidem tartrate (sedative)

gastrointestinal anti-spasmodics prescribed for irritable bowel or ulcer such as hyoscyamine (Anaspaz, ED-SPAZ, Gastrosed, Levsin)

sulfonylureas drugs for control of Type II diabetes (Diabinase, Orinase)

coal tar for skin and scalp conditions (Doak Tar Oil, Balnetar, Zetar Emulsioin, Polytar Bath)

oral contraceptives (estrogen/progestin combinations)

minoxidil for baldness (Rogaine)

antipsychotic drugs (phenothiazine, haloperidol)

eretinate, isoretinoin for skin problems (Retin-A)

## Drugs That Increase the Risk of Hemorrhage in the Eyes

The following drugs increase your risk of hemorrhage in the delicate vessels of the eye and elsewhere in the body:

pentoxifylline, used to relieve painful blood clotting

in the legs that can be a result of blood vessel disease (Trental)

other oral anticoagulants (heparin, coumadin, anisindione)

NSAIDs (ibuprofen, flurbiprofen, ketoprofen, naproxen)

venlafaxine (antidepressant)

cholinesterase inhibitors (prescribed for Alzheimer's disease)

amphotericin B (antibiotic)

## Drugs That Can Directly Damage the Retina

Hydroxychloroquine sulfate (Plaquenil), a drug prescribed for rheumatoid arthritis, has caused irreversible retinal damage in some patients. While using this drug, you must have frequent eye exams and be alert to any visual symptoms such as light flashes or streaks, which may be signs of retinal damage.

Other drugs that can damage the retina include:

thioridazine, an anti-infective drug that can cause pigmentary retinopathy

clonidine (Catapres), an alpha-adrenergic drug for lowering of blood pressure

NSAIDs

terbinafine, mefloquine (antibiotics)

## Drugs That Can Cause or Worsen Cataracts

glucocorticoids (Prednisone, cortisone)

NSAIDs

fluoroquinone, terbinafine, mefloquine (antibiotic)

eretinate, isoretinoin (for skin disorders)

## Drugs That Can Cause or Worsen Glaucoma or Damage the Optic Nerve

glucocorticoids

simvastatin

fenfluramine

NSAIDs

mirtazapine (antidepressant)

venlafaxine

gastrointestinal antispasmodics for ulcer and irritable bowel syndrome such as (Hyoscyamine Anaspaz, ED-SPAZ, Donnamar, Gastrosed, Levsin, Levbid)

hyoscyamine sulfate

## Drugs That Can Cause Blood Clotting, Impeding Blood Flow to the Eyes

estrogen (Premarin for example)

Androgen replacement with synthetic hormones (methyltestosterone, fluoxymetosterone)

## Other Visual Side Effects of Prescription Drugs

Changes in visual sharpness, conjunctivitis, dry eye, itchy eyes, corneal abrasion, and double vision are a few of the problems you may encounter while using prescription medications. Even the drops used for eye problems such as glaucoma and dry eye can cause discomfort and impair vision temporarily. Because so many prescription drugs have ocular side effects that go away when the drug is discontinued, we won't try to list them all here. It's important for you to know that your eye problems could be improved significantly by weaning yourself off prescription medications. This is a good reason to read your drug information insert carefully, even if you have to get out a magnifying glass to do it.

Please don't stop taking any medication "cold turkey" without first checking with your doctor, and don't stop taking a prescription drug without consulting a health care professional. Some powerful drugs have significant side effects that need to be controlled with additional medications. If you must take medication, support your body with good nutrition, exercise, and supplements.

## Overprescribed Drugs That Are Best Avoided for Long-Term Eye Health

**Corticosteroids** such as prednisone are probably the worst culprits when it comes to eye damage caused by drugs. These medications are used to control inflammation in the body and to treat autoimmune diseases, arthritis, asthma, and skin disorders. You may be prescribed steroid eye drops after surgery. Steroid drugs can make you more vulnerable to fungal eye infection and can mask the infection's symptoms. If you must use a corticosteroid drug, be sure to take high doses of antioxidants (vitamins C, E, and beta-carotene, among others) to help prevent steroid-induced cataracts.

Sometimes a small dose of hydrocortisone, a natural cortisone, rather than higher doses of the synthetics such as prednisone can do the job without the side effects. It's worth asking if you feel you must be taking steroids.

**NSAIDs such as aspirin, ibuprofen, and acetaminophen** are commonly used drugs in both over-the-counter and prescription varieties. Photosensitivity, damage to the gastrointestinal tract, dry eyes, corneal deposits, liver impairment, and cataracts can all result from use of NSAIDs.

**Antibiotics** have saved countless lives and all but eradicated some infectious diseases. Now, doctors hand out prescriptions for antibiotics even if they aren't sure they are needed. Just like those household pests that become resistant to pesticides, antibiotic-resistant strains of bacteria evolve and render these miracle drugs useless in some instances. Antibiotics disrupt the body's balance; the more you use them the less likely they are to work effectively when you need them. Antibiotics often cause photosensitivity, gastrointestinal difficulties, and changes in liver function. They suppress your own immune function. Vitamin C in high doses and probiotics such as acidophilus or bifidus are musts during antibiotic therapy. In our experience, those who care for themselves well and stay on their supplement plans very rarely need antibiotics at all.

**Diuretics** are another overprescribed class of drugs that can wreak havoc with the delicately balanced systems that regulate fluid volume in the body. Draining the body of fluid to lower blood pressure is a classic example of treating a symptom rather than the cause. Temporary use of diuretics to bring down very high blood pressure may be useful while you're making necessary lifestyle changes, but nutrition, supplements, and exercise are vastly more effective and healthier in the long run because they get at the underlying cause of the problem.

### IN SHORT . . .

1.  Avoid taking prescription or over-the-counter drugs whenever possible. Instead, use healthy lifestyle measures and good nutrition to prevent disease and treat ill health.

2.  Know the various effects and side effects that any drugs you take could have on your vision, and try to eliminate or reduce their use if you know they could impact your eyesight in a negative way.

3.  If you have to use prescription or over-the-counter drugs, know both their generic names and their brand names, know their effects and side effects, know how they interact with other drugs, and record which you use on a list to travel with you everywhere so that in an emergency the people who care for you will know what may be in your system and adjust their treatment accordingly.

4.  Many drugs interfere with the absorption and transport of nutrients. Know what they are and try to adjust your drug regimen to avoid those that are harmful in this manner. Take vitamins and supplement your diet with healthy foods if you must take such drugs so that your eyes, as well as the other

parts of your body, are not cheated of good nutrition.

5. Common drugs to lower blood pressure and cholesterol can spell trouble for your eyes. And many drugs cause photosensitization; your eyes will need protection from the sun, just as your skin does, during the use of such pharmaceuticals.

6. Some drugs specifically can cause eye problems such as clotting, optic nerve damage, hemorrhage, dryness, et cetera. Know what they are and try to avoid them.

7. Many common over-the-counter or prescription drugs such as NSAIDs and antibiotics can harm the eye. Live without them if possible.

# 12

## Exercise Your Way to Clear Vision

Your body is designed for movement and activity. Walking, climbing, bending, stretching, lifting, and frolicking are as natural as your heartbeat or breathing. The way our lives are structured these days tends to make it difficult to indulge our desires to move. After years of being stuck at desks and in cars, that instinct can fade. Suddenly exercise seems like work. We need special clothes and shoes and a membership to a gym. Hundreds of books and magazines are devoted to how best to exercise. It's easy to forget that after all, our bodies already know how to move. Unless you're ill or injured, or have been sedentary for years, you can start your exercise program right now by getting up and going for a walk.

You probably know somebody who's a self-described fitness freak, for whom anything less than a ten-mile run over hilly terrain is not a workout. The guy who prides himself on having a biceps muscle as big around as your head, or the woman who spends three hours a day at the gym and has the figure of a young boy might make you wonder if you're doing enough. We would like to encourage you to avoid those kinds of extremes (see step 2 in Chapter 1, "Everything in moderation"). Sooner or later we pay for going to extremes, and they are contrary to good sense and good health.

You'll be glad to know that anything that involves movement counts as exercise. George Burns lived to be one hundred and his exercise regimen consisted of doing his own housework. Gardening, window shopping, carrying groceries or laundry, and playing with children all count as exercise.

As a general rule, all that's needed to gain significant health benefits is light to moderate physical activity for thirty minutes a day. Those thirty minutes don't have to be consecutive; they can be broken up into fifteen-, ten-, or even five-minute segments throughout the day.

Remember that something is always better than nothing. If you're inactive now, you can get a lot out of simply becoming more active. Walking from the far end of the parking lot, taking the stairs instead of the elevator, or doing household chores to music is a great beginning to a more active lifestyle. If you do adopt a more structured program of exercise, you should still try to incorporate more activity into your daily routine.

If you have been diagnosed with high blood pressure, heart disease, diabetes, or lung disease, you should check with a health care professional before you get started. There may be special guidelines you need to follow, or your health care professional might recommend you have a treadmill test where you can be carefully monitored as you exercise. If you're taking any prescription drugs, you should check with your doctor or pharmacist to see whether they will affect how your body responds to exercise.

A diet lacking in nutrition doesn't give you much "get up and go," but it can give you far more calories than you need, making you one of millions of people fighting the battle of the bulge. Weight loss is no less than an obsession in this country, and the desire to drop extra pounds is the primary reason people get started with exercise.

Getting some exercise isn't only about how you look, though; obesity is linked to higher risk of heart disease, adult-onset diabetes, high blood pressure, and orthopedic problems, and it's certainly linked to eye disease.

Exercise, especially the aerobic or cardiovascular variety, is one of the most important things you can do to improve your body's ability to circulate blood filled with nutrients and oxygen through the vessels. Every bout of exercise pushes the circulatory system to do its job more efficiently. Over time this brings the body to a higher level of function overall.

Combined with the dietary changes we've described in this book, daily exercise will certainly help you to lose weight. We want you to know, though, that being thin at any cost is a lot unhealthier than carrying a few extra pounds. Recent research has shown very clearly that if you exercise, you will enjoy improved health, whether or not you lose any weight at all. It's not smart or sensible to attempt to maintain the body you had when you were in your twenties when you're in your forties, fifties, or sixties. It won't work, and you'll put yourself through a lot of stress worrying about it.

However, the old adage of "use it or lose it" is never more true than with exercise, and is especially true as we age. Joints, muscles, and circulatory systems that don't move get painful, weak, leaky, and creaky! Movement, on the other hand, keeps the body strong, resilient, and better able to resist disease and deterioration.

It's never too late to begin exercising. We don't care how long it's been since you've taken a walk or how old you are, you will benefit the instant you get up and get moving. If you've been sedentary, begin slowly and be gentle with yourself. If you experience pain, that's feedback from your body that you're overdoing it. Listen carefully to these signals and back off. The next time you exercise, you'll be able to do more.

Arthritis is not a reason to avoid exercise. In fact, both osteoarthritis and rheumatoid arthritis respond very well to gentle exercise. Study after study has shown that people who get some exercise experience less arthritis pain and take less pain medication than their sedentary counterparts. And by the way, exercise is also a great way to prevent these painful diseases.

## What Type of Exercise Is Best for You?

Your best criterion for what type of exercise is best for you is whether you enjoy it. When you enjoy exercise, you'll make it a regular part of your life. Even the most sophisticated exercise routine won't work if you don't do it. If you enjoy a yoga or qi gong class but hate aerobic exercise, then just be grateful that you enjoy the yoga and do that. If you love a good heart-pounding run on the treadmill but find yoga boring, then go for the treadmill. If you can't get yourself to move unless you're playing with or against someone else, go for it. If a walk around the block is all you can manage, fine!

If you have the time and energy, you can fine-tune your exercise regimen, but we certainly don't want you to be concerned if you're not doing every type of exercise mentioned here. Any effort you make will have a positive effect on your health. Be guided by a sense of enjoyment rather than a sense of duty.

People start exercise programs over and over and never can seem to stick with them. It's usually because they think it's all or nothing, and they start into a program so gung-ho that they get burned out in a matter of weeks. When exercise is a natural part of your life, you will be one step closer to the vitality and clarity you're striving for.

The greatest benefits of exercise are seen in those who have been completely sedentary "couch potatoes" and who start a program of light to moderate activity. It doesn't have to be painful, you don't have to sweat buckets, you don't have to suffer from muscle soreness or stitches in your sides. Just get moving!

Here's a quick guide to different types of exercise.

**Aerobic exercise** isn't just what you get in an aerobics class. It's any kind of physical activity that makes your heart beat faster, also known as raising your heart rate. As you move the large muscle groups in your arms, legs, and trunk, more blood flows faster through your vessels to "feed" the working muscles. Walking, jogging, cycling, cross-country skiing, swimming, and dancing are all forms of aerobic exercise.

**Resistance exercise** involves working various muscles against resistance. You can use dumbbells, weight machines, rubber tubing, cans of food, other household items, or your own body weight to provide resistance. Push-ups, biceps curls, leg lifts, yoga exercises, and squatting are examples of resistance exercises.

As we age, our body composition changes. That means that we lose muscle and gain fat with passing years. The good news is that you can keep much of the muscle you had in your youth with resistance training. If you challenge your muscles to the point of fatigue two or three times a week, using dumbbells, rubber tubing, or the machines at the gym, you can convince your body that it needs to keep muscle that might otherwise break down from disuse. Those who maintain muscle strength as they age have fewer falls, thanks to greater strength and better balance.

Fat can be reduced by increasing muscle mass because muscle is a calorie-burner that consumes calories from food that might otherwise go directly to your fat cells. Even while you're at rest that extra muscle you've built with resistance training is burning up calories just to maintain itself. Resistance training also helps to strengthen connective tissues like tendons and ligaments, making them less vulnerable to injury.

**Stretching, also known as flexibility training,** involves gentle holding and pushing into poses designed to lengthen muscle and connective tissue. It's best to do these exercises when your body is warmed up, so that your muscles are more pliable.

Flexibility is an important part of fitness. If you don't work to keep your joints supple, imbalances can occur in your body as a result of muscle and connective-tissue tightness. For example, chronic low back pain often occurs because of tightness in the hamstrings (the big muscles that run down the back of your thigh) that tips your pelvis under, changing the natural curved position of your lower spine. Your back wasn't meant to be pulled this way.

Yoga, an ancient Asian form of exercise, incorporates flexibility training with breathing, meditation, and relaxation exercises. Taking time each day to meditate by focusing on your breathing, perhaps sitting against a wall or lying on your back, will do wonders for your well-being. Qi gong and Tai Chi are Asian movement systems that stretch the body in a series of gentle, graceful movements.

## The Benefits of Exercise

With regular exercise your body gains many benefits:

✓ Your heart gets stronger and can pump more blood with each beat. As a result, your heart has less work to do to nourish your body adequately. Your resting heart rate goes down after a month or so of regular exercise.

✓ Circulation is improved, and that means better blood flow to your eyes.

✓ Daily tasks that once tired you out aren't as difficult anymore. You have a lot more energy and strength.

✓ The quality of your sleep will improve dramatically as soon as you start to exercise regularly.

✓ Weight-bearing aerobic exercise like walking, stair-climbing, or lifting weights keeps bones strong and resistant to osteoporosis.

✓ Your immune system is fortified and can better fight infection when you stick with a workout program.

✓ Breathing becomes deeper and more efficient.

✓ Good (HDL) cholesterol gets a boost and blood triglycerides (fats) are reduced.

✓ High blood pressure can be controlled with regular exercise.

✓ Diabetics can reduce the amount of insulin they have to use.

IN SHORT . . .

1. In order to gain substantial health bene-fits, add up thirty minutes of physical activity on most days of the week. Anything that gets you up and moving counts!

2. The health of your eyes is dependent on good circulation. The benefits of being more active include improved cir-culation throughout the body, better sleep, heightened mood, stronger immunity to infection, and more endurance.

3. High blood pressure, diabetes, and breathing problems all can be signifi-cantly improved with regular exercise.

4. Aerobic exercise, resistance training, flexibility, and stress reduction all should be addressed in an optimal exercise program.

# 13

## How to Avoid Vision-Destroying Toxins and Cleanse Your Body of Them

Living in civilization certainly has its advantages. We live in great comfort, in buildings that can be carefully climate-controlled, with plush carpeting, stain-resistant furniture, and attractive paneling. Eliminating bothersome pests is as easy as a visit from the exterminator. We can travel over long distances easily, in planes and cars as comfortable as our homes. We can go to the grocery store and buy processed foods that require minimal preparation, saving us significant time and energy. There's no denying it, we've got it pretty good.

Our standard of living comes with a price, however. Our comfortable homes are likely also hazardous to our health because of toxic chemicals in carpets, furniture, and paneling. Air conditioning and heating ducts grow filthy and recirculate debris, molds, and fungus into your home. Those pesticides and herbicides designed to kill critters in your home and yard are toxic to you as well. Cars, planes, and factories pollute the air we breathe. Meats and cheeses cooked at very high temperatures produce carcinogens. Food additives and artificial sweeteners may make food preparation easier, but aren't as harmless as we've been led to believe.

There is growing concern about the effects of environmental toxins on our health. The established mainstream medical community is encountering more and more patients who are most definitely sick, but for whom they can't come up with a diagnosis. These unfortunate people get sent home with a list of prescription drugs to treat their headaches, fatigue, muscle aches, depression, irritable bowel, or rashes. Symptoms might be alleviated temporarily but return as soon as medication is stopped. Side effects from the medications complicate things further.

Practitioners of naturopathic medicine have long maintained that toxins in the body can cause illness. The root causes of degenerative diseases (such as rheumatoid arthritis) and cancers have been traced to the accumulation of these toxins beyond the body's capacity for neutralizing them. We predict that as diagnoses of environmental illness, multiple chemical sensitivity, and multiple allergy become more common in the offices of medical doctors, a merging of the age-old art of cleansing the body of toxins with more mainstream treatments may be the only way for doctors trained in traditional medicine to help these patients. Environmental health is too crucial an issue for mainstream physicians to continue to ignore. Physicians and patients both will benefit as medical doctors learn more about the use of nutrition and herbal remedies for bolstering the body's own detoxification systems.

Obviously it isn't practical for you to try to avoid all potential toxins. We don't want you to live in a hermetically sealed bubble. What you can do is maximize your body's formidable defense systems and avoid major toxin loads whenever possible. Occasional cleansing of the body by fasting, sweating in a sauna, and herbal and nutritional therapies will benefit you a great deal by purging and neutralizing stored-up toxins.

Chelation therapy, which involves the infusion of a man-made protein known as *ethylenediaminetetraacetic acid* (EDTA) into your bloodstream in a doctor's office, is a reliable way to clear your body of toxic heavy metals. It has been used successfully in treatment of artery disease and health problems caused by heavy metal toxicity. We know doctors who prescribe it to their patients with macular degeneration, and they report that it helps slow the progress of the disease and in some cases even improves vision.

The following are the major categories of toxic substances to be aware of and avoid whenever possible.

## Chemical Toxins

Chemical toxins include pesticides, herbicides, formaldehyde (in insulation, plywood, and the polyurethane foam in pillows, cushions, and mattresses, and under rugs), oil vapors, household chemicals such as those used in cleaning supplies, tobacco smoke, ozone from electrical appliances, chlorinated/fluoridated water, polyesters, polyethylene plastics, food additives (preservatives, buffers, stabilizers, colorings, and flavorings), and fillers used in the making of medicines. Injury by these man-made chemicals happens at the cellular level, as cells' metabolic machinery is "gunked up" by the foreign substances. Chemical damage can lead to an increased free-radical load, which also causes damage to cells.

## Keep Your Brain Free of Excitotoxins

What do MSG, short for monosodium glutamate, and aspartame, also known by its trade names NutraSweet and Equal, have in common? Both are food additives used to make processed foods more palatable to the taste buds of consumers. Both contain *excitotoxins*—natural amino acids that stimulate brain cells. In the body, levels of aspartic acid (one of the breakdown components of aspartame) and glutamine (a main ingredient of monosodium glutamate) are tightly regulated. A little bit of coffee will wake you up gently, but an entire pot will give you a serious case of the jitters. In the same way, the precise quantity and balance of excitotoxins normally found in the brain maintains brain function, while too much literally excites cells to death.

Soft drinks are the biggest source of aspartame consumption. Its most common side effects include headaches (by far the most common complaint), memory loss, foggy thinking, irritability, itching, ringing ears, and (believe it or not) weight gain. Aspartame also contains methanol, or wood alcohol. Methanol is a known retinal and optic nerve toxin. Vision problems and dry eyes are among the complaints the FDA often hears about aspartame. No less than 78 percent of the complaints to the Food and Drug Administration in 1996 were regarding this purportedly "harmless" alternative to sugar!

Monosodium glutamate (MSG), widely used to enhance flavor in processed foods such as soups, chips, cereals, baked goods, and frozen foods contains the excitotoxin glutamate. It has been estimated that 30 percent of the population is allergic to MSG. Scientists are looking at possible connections between MSG and migraine headaches, asthma attacks, and rheumatoid arthritis. MSG is found in countless processed foods under a wide variety of names (see Chapter 9). Please do your best to avoid MSG and aspartame.

## Awash in a Sea of Hormones

Many petrochemicals (made from petroleum products) act as *xenobiotics*, or substances that actually mimic hormones in the body and interfere with the actions of our own hormones. Imagine standing at a locked door with a set of keys, all of which fit into the lock but only one of which opens the door. Think of the door as an important reaction in your body, and the body's natural hormone as the key that will open it. Xenobiotics are like the keys that simply take up the lock without opening it. That means you can't get into the room to do whatever you came there to do, and that's the problem with xenobiotic chemicals: The reaction the natural hormone is designed to complete doesn't happen if a fake version has taken its place. Some others, such as xenoestrogens, are many times more potent than the natural versions—in other words, they're keys of the James Bond ilk that will blow the door out of its hinges when inserted into the keyhole.

The vast majority of xenobiotics come from pesticides and plastics. Some of the most potent are by-products of manufacturing known as PCBs and dioxins. These are already widespread throughout the food chain and present in our fat cells. While they may not have immediate or dramatically negative effects on an adult, their effects on the unborn fetus, infants, and young children can be devastating.

## Keeping Free Radicals in Line

Free radicals (also known as *pro-oxidants*) are produced constantly in your body as it goes about the business of maintaining itself. As long as your antioxidant defenses are up to the task, free radicals are squelched before they can do you harm. If too heavy a load of chemical toxins exists, free-radical production increases dramatically. These reactive molecules then can target the fats in your blood or cell structures and transform them into lipid peroxides, which can contribute to heart disease and other chronic diseases. Heavy metals (discussed in the next section) are especially problematic creators of free radicals. Free radicals also can alter proteins and DNA, setting the stage for cancer and possibly autoimmune diseases such as rheumatoid arthritis and irritable bowel syndrome.

## Be Wary of Heavy Metals

Heavy metals such as lead, cadmium, arsenic, nickel, and aluminum are much more plentiful in our environment than ever before. Daily exposure to trace amounts of these metals can add up to dangerous accumulation in the body. Did you know about these sources of heavy metals you encounter every day?

**Lead:** Water (leaches from lead pipes), some plastics, electric cable insulation, gasoline additives, insecticides, pigments in the paint that flakes off your walls and becomes dust that you breathe, newsprint, pottery glaze, and porcelain enamel.

**Aluminum:** Antacids, douches, antidiarrheal agents, physician-prescribed anti-ulcer remedies, buffered aspirins, processed food products such as cheeses, baking powder, cake mixes, and cookware.

**Mercury:** Mainly from dental fillings. There's considerable support for the hypothesis that mercury amalgam fillings can cause Alzheimer's disease.

Some types of fish, especially swordfish, are contaminated with mercury. Grains and produce are grown from seeds often treated with mercury fungicide. This extremely toxic metal is also found in some fabric softeners, adhesives, and floor waxes, and it is a common contaminant in industrial areas.

The point is, you don't have to work in a factory to have unsafe levels of heavy-metal buildup in your body. It's around you every day.

Heavy metals do damage by interfering with enzyme systems and shutting down important antioxidant defenses. Free radicals then can run rampant, doing damage from the cell level to the DNA level. As you have read earlier, in Chapter 2 and throughout this book, free radicals are one of the leading causes of damage to the eyes.

## Who's Protecting Us from Toxins?

If these toxic substances are so dangerous, you ask, why are some of them so readily available? Why are they in our homes, in our offices and cars, in the very medications our doctors prescribe to make us well? Why is everyone saying that they are safe to use? *One-quarter million* new substances are introduced into the environment each year. It's impossible to verify the safety of each one with thorough scientific studies. Even if that were possible, the testing of a single chemical doesn't give us any idea of how it will interact with the thousands of other chemicals it would encounter in your body.

The majority of the tens of thousands of chemicals used in products you use in your home have not been studied. Their effects on your health are unknown. It takes a couple of generations of exposure to a chemical before we have a good grasp of its potential for harm. Some chemicals seem to do no damage until the babies of exposed parents are deformed or have poor reproductive or mental function. The Food and Drug Administration (FDA) tests new products and awards them the GRAS (Generally Recognized as Safe) label if their testing does not reveal cancer-causing or other harmful properties, but the procedures for testing aren't thorough enough to catch all potential problems.

Plenty of drugs have been tested and labeled as GRAS, only to be recalled later, after causing enormous harm, again often to the children of exposed parents. Food additives such as benzoic acid, sulfites, nitrites, BHA, and BHT are GRAS, but their safety is being called into question years after their use began.

Don't underestimate, either, the influence of economics. Chemical companies are huge and wealthy. Their main interest is in making money, and they pay scientists handsomely if they can prove that their latest cleaning solvent is as harmless as a bouquet of carnations. Any attempt by the government to regulate more strictly the manufacture and sale of toxic chemicals is met by great resistance from those with a vested interest in the chemical industry. When it comes down to election time, it's nice to have those big boys on your side.

It's beyond the scope of this book to go into detail on this very important topic, but if you're interested in learning more, we've supplied you with a list of recommended readings in Appendix II. These books will describe in detail how these harmful materials have accumulated in the environment over the past century, and how to steer clear of toxic chemicals and heavy metals wherever possible, especially in your home.

Our emphasis as doctors, given the incontrovertible fact that you have had lifelong exposure to toxins, is on how to periodically cleanse your body so that the effects will not have a chance to accumulate. Your eye health, as well as the health of your entire body, will benefit from periodic cleansing. As you learned in Chapters 9 and 10, you must have healthy circulatory and digestive systems in order to have healthy eyes. Damage from environmental toxins affects all of the organ systems of the body, but the blood vessels and intestines are particularly vulnerable, putting your eyes at risk.

## EDTA Chelation Therapy

EDTA is a protein component that when infused into the bloodstream one or two times a week for a total of twenty to thirty treatments can bring about remarkable cures from angina or leg pains due to blocked blood vessels. Norman E. Clarke, Sr., M.D., who administered chelation treatments during World War II for the treatment of heavy metal toxicity, discovered that men who had angina before the treatments no longer suffered from it following them. Since that time, the therapy has shown much promise as a way to flush arteries clean of athero-sclerotic blockages.

The medical establishment has not accepted chelation as a safe, reliable treatment of artery disease. Considerable conflict has gone on between the American Medical Association (AMA) and the small but strong group of physicians who support the use of chelation therapy.

The American College for Advancement in Medicine, or ACAM, is the professional organization pushing for more large-scale studies on chelation. No large-scale studies have been published about EDTA chelation's effectiveness in any of the major medical journals read by physicians. Much of the evidence that it works has come from those who have administered it and seen its almost miraculous effectiveness.

Consider this: A bypass surgery costs sixty thousand dollars and is covered by insurance. Angioplasty costs about fifteen thousand dollars and is also covered. These treatments are what you'd have to choose from if you arrived at the hospital with severe chest pains from angina. Chelation costs five thousand to seven thousand dollars (or less), not including "boosters," and is not covered by most insurance companies, due to its status as an "experimental treatment."

Bypass surgeries bring over four billion dollars into hospital coffers each year. If it were safe and effective, this wouldn't concern us, but in all but the sickest heart patients the risks of surgery outweigh the benefits. Some medical authorities claim that bypass is the best way to relieve uncontrolled angina pains. But it's a temporary fix: In one large study of bypass patients, 24 percent had angina pains within one year, and a whopping 40 percent had them by the sixth year. Complications from the surgery are very common.

When there are alternatives such as the lifestyle changes we have suggested in this book, which time and time again have shown impressive results for severely ill heart-disease patients without drugs or surgery, and chelation therapy, the huge number of bypasses performed in U.S. hospitals is no less than an outrage. Most people who submit to bypass surgery are not informed of their other options, and are simply told that if they don't have the open-heart surgery, they will die.

Those who have angioplasties don't fare too well, either. Pushing the walls of an artery open with a tiny balloon works to open a clog, but the vessel is likely to close back up quickly. There's no solid evidence that angioplasty has any value as anything but a "Band-Aid" approach to the problem.

Chelation cleans the blood vessels throughout the body. If you have a clog in one vessel, you've got clogs in others, and you need to get to the root of the problem. It's interesting to note that several people who were helped by chelation to overcome disease so severe that doctors insisted they have more expensive, invasive, and risky procedures took their insurers to court, and the insurance companies were ordered to pay.

## What Is Chelation Therapy?

You go to the doctor's office with something to read and a nutritious snack. A nurse seats you in a comfortable chair and places an intravenous drip into your arm. For about three hours, a solution of EDTA, distilled water, and vitamins and minerals slowly will be infused into your bloodstream. Halfway through, you'll need to have your snack to stave off low blood sugar, and you may need to urinate a couple of times during the treatment. You'll repeat this once or twice a week for a total of twenty to thirty treatments, and thereafter you'll probably have "booster" treatments once or twice a month.

## How Does Chelation Work?

One way in which chelation is known to work is by binding excess calcium in your blood, and removing it from where it may be incorporated into the plaques that block arteries. You may think of calcium as an important component of teeth and bones, and this is the role of 99 percent of the body's necessary calcium. The other 1 percent needed is involved in heartbeat, nerve transmission, muscle contraction, and balance of blood acidity. Such *essential* calcium is spared during EDTA, bound as it is to proteins that make it impossible for EDTA to grab that calcium. Unbound, *excess* calcium also exists in your body. It tends to be stored in the joints and along the walls of the blood vessels. The worse your artery health, the more excess calcium you have lining your arteries. Atherosclerotic lesions are cemented together with this bad ("metastatic") calcium. EDTA binds with this calcium and removes it, flushing it out of the body and allowing the plaques to dissolve.

A bonus of chelation therapy is that the parathyroid gland is stimulated to release hormones that also break down metastatic calcium deposits. As all of this goes on, recalcification of bone is also stimulated.

Chelation therapy also may work to reduce the production of free radicals. Heavy metals like lead, iron, and mercury are potent catalysts of free-radical reactions. They are *pro-oxidants* that encourage the formation of free radicals, which then can do damage to any of the body's structures. There is also some evidence that heavy metals accumulating in brain tissues over a lifetime contribute to Alzheimer's disease. There are reports that chelation therapy has restored health to people who were thought to be lost to this heartbreaking disease.

EDTA chelation makes your blood less likely to clot where it shouldn't. Unwanted blood clots cause strokes, heart attacks, and death of eye tissues. Those with the predisposing factors for heart attack (high blood pressure, high blood cholesterol, and insulin resistance, to name a few) also tend to have "stickier" blood.

Finally, chelation therapy can help prevent arterial spasm. This may have something to do with removal of excess calcium, or with the clearing-away of irritating deposits along the blood vessel walls. Spasm of arteries can block blood flow as effectively as a blood clot can.

## Chelation and Eye Health

How can chelation therapy help those with eye disease? Because of its reduction of free-radical formation, which has been implicated as a cause of macular degeneration, it can reduce the harmful effects of sunlight on the macula. It can keep clear of clogs the vital blood vessels that feed the eyes and help to diminish those clogs that have already built up. The most compelling support for the use of chelation in treating eye problems is in the stories of those who have experienced significant visual improvement with it. Often improved vision is a "side effect" experienced by those who undergo chelation treatment for heart disease. Remember, anything that improves circulation will improve eye health.

These days chelation is a low-risk procedure in the hands of a competent physician. Kidney toxicity has been an unfortunate result of infusions given too rapidly, but this hasn't happened for decades. All of those heavy metals being carried out of the body must pass through the kidneys, and only small doses can be handled at once. Any physician with ACAM's stamp of approval will administer the treatments carefully, and you will be monitored by a nurse at all times.

Regular chelation treatments must be coupled with the nutritional guidelines in this book, regular exercise, and extra supplementation of vitamins (especially $B_6$), magnesium, and other minerals that can be depleted by chelation.

If you decide to try chelation, you can write or call ACAM (check Appendix II at the back of the book) to find out which doctors in your area are using this treatment.

## Fasting

Rats who are regularly deprived of food live longer than those fed every day. Food restriction slows cancer growth. It is well established that rats benefit greatly from fasting, which means going without food. We think it would be safe to say that the majority of alternative health care professionals also find it beneficial to have their patients fast occasionally. We're not talking here about extreme deprivation, we're talking about giving your body a break.

As we've already said, there's no way to completely avoid exposure to toxins. There are simply too many of them. But you can take steps to prevent them from accumulating beyond your capacity to buffer or eliminate them. Unexplainable nausea, headache, tiredness, joint pains, or muscle aches are good indicators that your buffering and elimination systems are being overwhelmed.

During a fast the body has a chance to metabolize stored wastes and toxins so that they can be flushed out. The digestive system gets to take a breather, as stomach acid, pepsin, and pancreatic enzyme secretion falls. Freedom from the gut damage due to food allergens allows the gut linings to heal. Avoid heavy exercise when you're fasting and try taking saunas (guidelines appear at the end of this chapter) to aid the elimination of toxins through the skin. Relaxing, sunbathing, massage, and gentle stretching exercises can be beneficial during a fast.

Classic fasting with nothing but water for four days isn't advisable for anyone suffering from ill health unless you are under the supervision of a health care professional experienced in this area. A modified version of the water fast is a program called Ultra Clear Plus (HealthComm), put together by Jeff Bland, Ph.D. The use of a nutrient-dense powder mixed with pure water helps you to maintain your energy levels throughout the fast while still enjoying the benefits of fasting. The kit, which you can buy at most health food stores, will give you complete instructions.

You can also go on a juice fast, just drinking organic, unfiltered apple or pear juice three to four times a day. Even a vegetable juice fast is beneficial, but use bland vegetables such as carrots and beets (not too many, they're very sweet) and celery. We recommend that in a juice fast you mix one tablespoon of psyllium powder with your juice (at least an eight-ounce glass), and follow that with a glass of water, when you normally would have a meal. This gives the intestines something to work on and doesn't stop their movement. Some people advocate shutting down the intestines, but then you have to get them started again, and that can be problematic.

Although a longer fast will cleanse the body more quickly and thoroughly, we recommend the less extreme alternatives. Our pursuit of moderation even extends to fasting! A three-to-five-day fast will give you many benefits, especially if you begin and end it with a few days of eating only brown rice, steamed vegetables, and salads. Here are some variations on the theme:

**Cleansing diet:** Eat only organic fruits and vegetables for all of a day's meals. Do this once or twice a week. Drink plenty of water.

**One-day fluid fast:** Go twenty-four to thirty-six hours with only water, vegetable broth (make some yourself), herb tea, and fruit and vegetable juices. You can use a meal replacement powder such as Ultra Clear if you get lightheaded from low blood sugar, although fruit juices should keep your blood sugar up.

If these fasts feel comfortable to you, you can try them for two or three days at a time. Taper your food intake gradually over the two to three days preceding the fast. Reintroduce your regular foods slowly once it's over, chewing everything thoroughly and eating small portions.

During a fast you can expect to have some unpleasant symptoms such as rashes, mucus discharge from the sinuses, cough, fatigue, moodiness, body odor, vision or hearing disturbances, or aches and pains. This happens as chemical toxins are released from stored fat into the bloodstream, and your body is reexposed to them. Break your fast immediately if you experience extreme weakness or dizziness, vomiting, diarrhea, or shortness of breath.

Your liver has to work hard to handle the increased flow of toxins during fasting, so you should be sure to take your vitamins and herbs diligently before you fast. You don't need to take them while you're fasting, but go right back to them after your fast is broken.

## Internal Cleansing with Nutritional Therapies

Your liver and your intestines are your most essential organs when it comes to internal cleansing. The liver is designed to filter out and neutralize toxic chemicals as they travel through the bloodstream. It's at risk, however, when the toxin load becomes too great for its many detoxification systems to handle effectively.

## Nutritional Prescription for Cleansing

Here are some nutritional guidelines you can follow before and after a fast to ensure that your liver is in tip-top shape. You can add the vitamins to our multivitamin recommendations. You can also use these supplements when you know you've been overexposed to toxins.

Vitamin C: up to 3 g (3,000 mg) in divided doses

Selenium: 100–200 mcg

Beta-carotene: up to 25,000 IU in divided doses

Milk thistle: 120 mg, 3 times in capsules; or 2 droppersful of the tincture in water, 3 times

Green tea (for its bioflavonoids called catechins): 2 cups

Glutathione-builders like N-acetyl cysteine, garlic, onions, eggs, and asparagus

Cruciferous family foods such as cabbage, broccoli, and brussels sprouts to stimulate liver function

Dandelion root: 4 g dried root; or 4–8 ml of fluid extract

*Taraxicum officionale*, 3 times to increase the flow of bile

Turmeric: as a spice, or 300 mg curcumin 3 times

Don't take benzodiapines (Prozac, Valium, Centrax, Librium, Ativan) or NSAIDs (aspirin, ibuprofen, acetaminophen). And don't drink more than one alcoholic beverage per day.

## Saunas

Twenty to thirty minutes in the sauna at 103–105 degrees Fahrenheit brings toxins out through the skin. If at any time you begin to feel nauseous, light-headed, faint, or dizzy, cut your sauna short. As soon as you leave the sauna, you should take a shower. Use a washcloth or natural sponge and soap (glycerine or Dr. Bronner's soaps are good choices) and scrub the entire body. You don't want to give those toxins a chance to be reabsorbed.

### IN SHORT . . .

1.  We are surrounded by toxins—
    chemicals in household cleaners,
    polyurethane foam in pillows, fillers in
    medicines, sugar substitutes that con-
    tain excitotoxins and can negatively
    affect your brain, and so on. Know your
    environment and reduce toxins if possi-
    ble for the health of your whole body,
    including your eyes.
2.  Xenobiotics, which mimic hormones,
    interfere with the natural action of our
    own hormones. Avoid the petrochemi-
    cals (usually plastics and pesticides) that
    contain xenobiotics.
3.  Free-radical production is boosted to an
    unhealthy level by chemical toxins,
    especially heavy metals such as lead
    and mercury. Try to rid your environ-
    ment of them—from your pipes, the
    paint on your walls, your dental fillings,
    and so on.
4.  Consider trying EDTA chelation therapy,
    which has many benefits for the eyes:
    reduced blood clotting, for one. (See
    the "Resources" section, Appendix I, for
    more information.)
5.  Try a fast or modified fast to cleanse
    your body. Sauna sessions also can rid
    your body of toxins, which can only
    help your vision.

# 14

# Basic Eye Care

So far you've learned about ways to improve your eye health and your vision by taking measures to improve your whole-body health. In this chapter we're going to give you some practical tips on eye care. You'll find out about which sunglasses are best for your particular eye problems and how to use eye drops so they help your eyes instead of harming them. We'll also give you some solutions for dry eyes and irritation caused by eye allergies.

## Sunglasses

Been to the beach lately? Sunbathers are still flocking there to expose as much skin to the sun's rays as they possibly can. Many of them use sunscreen now because of the public's growing awareness that sun exposure increases skin cancer risk and accelerates skin aging. Their eyes are usually shaded by sunglasses—another wise move, you might think. Sunglasses are as necessary a part of sun protection as that SPF 30 you rub onto your skin. Right?

Right . . . but the sunglasses those beachgoers are wearing are probably doing vastly more harm than good. If sunglasses don't block out 100 percent of ultraviolet radiation (UV-A and UV-B rays), they aren't doing much to protect your eyes. Worse yet, the dark lenses that shade away some of the sun's brightness reduce the reflexive squinting that is your body's natural response to excessive light. You certainly will feel more comfortable with those sunglasses on, but you aren't protected from the ultraviolet rays that contribute to macular degeneration and cataracts.

The manufacturers of sunglasses aren't closely regulated, so millions of pairs of useless sunglasses are sold in stores, and up to 40 percent of these are mislabeled. As the ozone layer thins, scientists expect that skin cancers will become more and more common. What you don't hear about too often is the dramatic increase in cataract occurrence that also is expected with ozone depletion. Very little ultraviolet radiation strikes the retina because it has to pass through the yellowish sun-shield provided by the lens. Still, it takes only a minuscule amount to kill off retinal light-receptor cells. In older people who have cloudy cataracts removed, threat of macular degeneration rises. Those who have cataracts removed need to be especially careful to shield their eyes from ultraviolet rays.

Sun damage to the eyes tends to occur gradually over years of exposure, with slow breakdown of proteins in the lenses of the eyes, clouding of vision, and development of cataracts. During the first thirty years of life, the eyes are more transparent, and the irreplaceable retinal cells are at greater risk. Even young people need to be concerned with protecting their eyes from sun damage.

## Guidelines for Choosing Sunglasses

Choosing the right sun protection for your eyes is an important part of maintaining your vision. Here are some guidelines for you to follow, but the single most important factor is the first one on the list: Get sunglasses that filter out the UV rays.

- Lenses must block out 100 percent of UV-A and UV-B rays. Since so many sunglasses are mislabeled, you need to find out which ones really do the job with an ultraviolet light sensor. Optiwear sells its Ultraviolet Sensometer for only five dollars (Optiwear, 3100 James Street, Syracuse, NY 13206). With this gadget, you can take a pair of sunglasses outdoors and test them. Any UV rays that go through the lenses will cause the card to change color. This is a very small investment for your eye health, and you can carry it in your wallet.
- Don't be fooled into thinking that a darker lens indicates better protection. The darkness of sunglass lenses isn't related to their level of protection from ultraviolet radiation. Lighter-tinted lenses will give you better visibility.
- Sun goggles that cover a large area and include side shields are your best bet for total protection.

These are great for those who wear prescription glasses, as they can fit right over them comfortably. You'll also get protection from airborne eye irritants and allergens, and moisture won't evaporate from the eyes as quickly.

- Opt for lightweight plastic, shatterproof (polycarbonate) sunglasses if you are active in sports. A glare-reducing polarizing film can be used on glass lenses, but glass can be very heavy for daily wear and is not made into large sun goggles. Polarization helps you see better in very bright light but doesn't protect you from UV radiation.
- Lens color may vary. The most popular is grey because it doesn't affect color perception. Yellow lenses may help reduce night glare for those with cataracts. Orange-brown lenses are best for those with macular degeneration because UV and blue-light rays are filtered out, offering the best retinal protection. Blues and violets look grey through orange-brown lenses, which bothers some people. Green lenses are popular and give the wearer a natural view, because there isn't much distortion of color as there can be with other lens tints.
- Scratch-protected lenses resist scratching that often occurs during sunglass cleaning.
- Mirrored lenses may increase comfort but don't filter UV rays.
- In addition to your sunglasses, it's a good idea to wear a hat with at least a three-inch brim. This will shade your face and give you added eye protection.

- Blue light, which is part of the visible spectrum, reacts with pigment deposits on the retina to make free radicals. This causes retinal damage that can, over the years, result in macular degeneration and loss of central vision. Wear sunglasses that filter out at least some blue light. When you wear them outside, a blue sky will look grey.

---

### FACTS ABOUT ULTRAVIOLET RADIATION

- UV radiation doesn't cause you to feel pain in your eyes like the pain of sunburned skin.
- The UV-B and UV-A rays don't feel hot on the skin, as do other, less dangerous kinds of solar radiation.
- UV rays are just as hazardous on a cloudy day as on a sunny day. There is some added risk because people are unaware of the need for protection on cloudy days.
- UV-B rays, strongest between 10 A.M. and 2 P.M., are considered the most harmful. This form of radiation is the one responsible for the manufacture of vitamin D in your skin. Only a few minutes of exposure a day is necessary for this conversion.

---

# Eye Drops

Using eye drops can be very challenging as we age. Shaky hands, poor aim, arthritis that makes it difficult to squeeze tiny bottles, uncontrolled blinking, and problems reading labels affect up to half of older patients given eye drops. To make matters even worse, few doctors give adequate instructions to their patients when prescribing these medications.

The best way to use eye drops is to (1) pull down the lower lid with one hand and (2) squeeze the drops into the space between the lower lid and the eyeball. Look upward just before applying the drop. Do your best to avoid touching the tip of the dropper to any part of the eye or eyelid. Keep your eyes closed and shift your eyeballs so that it feels like you're looking down for a few minutes after the drops are in. Closing your eyes (not tightly) seals tear drains shut so that the medicine doesn't drain immediately off the eye. Don't rub or squeeze the eyelid. You also can gently pinch the inside corners of your eyes—this also helps keep tear drains closed so that medicine isn't wasted.

If the above method doesn't work, try the closed-eye technique, which is often recommended for administration of eye drops to children. This may require help from another person. Lie down and place the prescribed number of drops onto the inner corner of the eyelid, then open the eye so that the drops fall in. Close the eye again once the drops have entered it, and follow the instructions given for the open-eye method from that point on.

To protect your eyes from bacteria, always wash your hands before instilling eye drops. Don't rinse the dropper, and keep it out of contact with the eye. Take care not to touch the dropper to fingers or countertops.

If your eye drops sting, keep them refrigerated. The cold is soothing and briefly numbs the eyes so that discomfort is minimized.

If you are using any ointments, which commonly are prescribed after surgery to help the eye heal, use them *after* other eye medications in drop form because they will keep fluids from absorbing into the eyes if used initially. For effective administration of ointments, first warm the tube in your hand for a few minutes. The first time you use the medication, squeeze out the first half-inch or so because it may have dried out. Tilt your head back and gaze upward. Pull out the lower lid to form a pouch, and then place $1/4$–$1/2$ inch of ointment along the lower lid, being careful to squeeze the tube gently. Then, slowly release the eyelid and keep it closed for one to two minutes, rolling the eyeball in all directions. Keep in mind that temporary blurring will occur, so you may want to delay activities like driving for a while. Use a tissue to remove excess ointment from around the eye. If there is another ointment you need to use after the first one, wait at least ten minutes before applying it.

## Avoid Preservatives in Eye Drops

Preservatives used in eye drops actually may worsen the problem for which you use the drops in the first place. Benzalkonium chloride, often used in "artificial tears" for dry eyes, temporarily relieves symptoms but makes dry eyes worse over time. This preservative also is found in eye drops for glaucoma and causes the eyes to dry out more quickly than drops that don't contain it. While prescription glaucoma drops without benzalkonium chloride are not available, you do have a choice when it comes to the use of "artificial tears." Look for those that are preservative-free. Some examples of brand names are Refresh, Refresh Plus and Relief by Allergan, Tears Naturale and BION by Alcon, Aquasite by CIBA Vision Care, and a Vitamin A drop by Vision called VIVA Drops.

## Treating Dry Eyes

Millions of adults suffer from dry, itchy, red, burning eyes. Artificial tears sold over-the-counter offer only temporary relief. As you might have already guessed, dry eyes are usually symptoms of problems affecting the entire body. An exception to this rule might exist in some older people who have droopy lower eyelids, so that too much of the eye's surface area is exposed and eye fluids evaporate more easily.

Medications such as diuretics and anti-glaucoma eye drops (because they contain harmful preservatives) often promote dry eye problems. Diabetics, arthritics, and those with cancer commonly complain of dry eyes. The use of the artificial sweetener aspartame has been linked to dry eyes.

Poor nutrition and hormone imbalances are probably the major culprits in causing dry eyes: Lack of essential fatty acids, vitamin A, vitamin C, riboflavin, and vitamin $B_6$ affect the workings of the eyes' lubrication systems. Since dry eyes are most common in menopausal women, it's probably safe to assume the hormonal imbalance has to do with low estrogen or progesterone. Our guess is that it's probably caused by estrogen dominance: Even when estrogen is low, if there's no progesterone to balance it, there are symptoms of excess estrogen. We have noticed that women who begin using natural progesterone cream often report that their dry eyes have cleared up.

Dry eyes also can be caused by allergies, often to some ingredient in cosmetics. If you suddenly start suffering from dry eyes, take a careful inventory of any new skin care products, shampoos, conditioners, makeup, and other products you recently have started using. If you stop using the product and the dry eyes clear up, you've found the culprit.

## How Tears Protect Your Eyes

Tears aren't just for crying. A film of tears made of three layers protects your eyes. One is a lipid (fat) layer, the interface between the inner two layers and the environment. Because of the fat, water can't evaporate through it. The middle layer is mostly water, and the inner layer contains mucin, which helps to spread tears across the surface of the eyeball

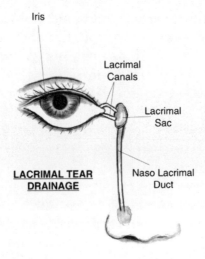

Iris

Lacrimal
Canals

Lacrimal
Sac

**LACRIMAL TEAR
DRAINAGE**

Naso Lacrimal
Duct

Blockage of the lacrimal glands or ducts of the eyes can cause dry eyes and irritation.

when you blink. Human tears also contain a special bacteria-killing enzyme to zap airborne bacteria.

Glands that secrete these oils, enzymes, and mucins are located in your eyelids. Blinking stimulates secretion from these glands. The lacrimal gland, located just below the brow, is responsible for the production of watery tears. Irritation from smoke, dust, wind, fumes, or smog triggers release of extra tears to moisten the eyes; strong emotions have the same effect (crying).

In people who suffer from autoimmune diseases such as rheumatoid arthritis, lupus, and childhood-onset diabetes, the lacrimal gland may shrivel and stop functioning. If the eyes lack oils and mucin, the lacrimal gland may work overtime to try to keep the eyes wet. People with this condition are surprised to find that the problem is actually *dry* eyes. Oversecretion of water dilutes the oils and mucin further.

If you have dry eyes, there are simple ways to restore the integrity of the tear film that keeps water against the eyeball rather than allowing it to evaporate. Omega-6 fatty acids help to restore the lipid layer. Use borage, black currant seed, or evening primrose oil. Omega-3 fatty acids from fish oil are also helpful. To improve the utilization of these fats in the body, take 50 mg of vitamin $B_6$ with them.

Vitamin A is an integral part of the mucin layer. Carrots, yams, sweet potatoes, and cantaloupes contain plentiful beta-carotene, which can be converted into vitamin A. Fish liver oil contains both omega-3 fatty acids and vitamin A, so eat plenty of fish. I also recommend preservative-free vitamin A drops. We recommend VIVA eyedrops, which you can ask for at your pharmacy.

Vitamin C also helps improve dry eye problems. There's a very high concentration of vitamin C in the natural tear film on the eyes, and eye irritants that cause the eyes to water dilute this antioxidant on the eyes' surface.

Drink plenty of pure water to improve the aqueous (watery) layer of the tear film. Avoid drinking too much coffee because its diuretic effect can worsen dry eye problems.

The following medications can cause eye dryness:

Antihistamines (Benadryl, Coricidin)

Atropine (a heart medication)

Any kind of diuretic (for high blood pressure)

Decongestants

Decongestant eye drops (Visine, Murine, ClearEyes, Prefrin)

Diazepam, Valium, Elavil (anti-anxiety drugs)

Methotrexate and other cancer drugs (chemotherapeutic agents)

Morphine

Niacin (used to treat high cholesterol)

Glaucoma eye drops (Betagan, Ocupress)

In stubborn cases of dry eyes or cases that involve damage to the cornea, you can take supplemental glucosamine sulfate. This natural substance, part of your body's pathway for building connective tissue, helps to build the collagen matrix of the cornea. Follow the directions on the bottle or take 500 mg three times a day.

Please don't try to instill herbal remedies or homemade eye drops into dry eyes. Eye drops should closely match the pH of the eye fluid. Anything too acidic will burn the eye. Be careful to keep eye drops separated from other similar-looking bottles, such as those containing glue or other household chemicals. Patients can put all kinds of things into their eyes, intentionally or unintentionally, and it can take some medical heroics to fix them up afterwards.

You can conserve moisture on the eyes by blinking more frequently, avoiding smog and fumes, and avoiding eye makeup (or reducing the amount you use). Check the nose pads of your glasses to be sure they don't pull the lower eyelids off the eyeballs. If you use a computer, set the monitor lower and tilt the screen up so that you can look down slightly, keeping the eyes narrowed. Humidifiers can be helpful for those with dry eyes.

There is a procedure called punctal occlusion that can help those with dry eyes who don't respond to nutritional changes. A tiny silicone plug is inserted into the tear drain at the inside lower corner of the eye. This prevents fluid from draining too quickly off the eye's surface and keeps the eyes moist. Your eye doctor may try temporary plugs that dissolve after a few days. If these work well, permanent plugs can be inserted. Laser surgery or cauterization also can be used to close the fluid drains. Plugging of the tear drains can help make contact lens wear more comfortable, reduce side effects from glaucoma eye drops (by keeping them in the eye rather than allowing them to drain), and even relieve postnasal drip or sinus problems.

Artificial tear inserts can also be used. These are small pellets of hydroxypropyl cellulose (sold under the trade name Lacrisert), which are inserted into the lower eyelid. They absorb fluid, swell up, and then release a nonmedicated moistening agent into the eye for twenty-four hours. These, like the tear drain plugs, are only for cases of dry eye that don't get better with the nutritional changes we've suggested.

During sleep, your eyes don't secrete tears. Blinking is your body's stimulus for tear secretion.

When you stop blinking, tear-producing glands take a rest. Those people whose eyes don't close completely during sleep have a condition known as lagophthalmos. Proteins build up over the exposed part of the eye during sleep, protecting it from drying out. Most people have small bits of this dried protein in the corners of their eyes when they wake up. If you have very stringy strands of mucus between your eyelids in the morning or if you often have trouble opening your eyes when you wake because the lids are stuck shut by these caked proteins, mention this to your eye doctor. He or she may recommend you tape your eyes closed when you go to sleep.

## Treating Eye Allergies

An allergy is the body's overreaction to a substance it labels as harmful. For example: What harm could the droppings of dust mites that live in furniture, bedding, clothing, and carpets do to the human body? The mites themselves are microscopic. Yet their tiny droppings are one of the most potent allergenic substances we know. People who are allergic to dust mites, pollen, animal dander, and other irritants suffer from sneezing, wheezing, itchy, watering eyes, and overproduction of mucus. Eyes swell, noses run continuously, and the skin may break out in itchy welts (hives). These reactions are caused by the release of inflammatory substances in the body in response to allergens.

Allergic eyes are itchy, watery, and often swollen. The overflow of water from the lacrimal glands dilutes the other components necessary to keep your eyes moist, and so allergic eyes are usually also dry at times. Eye doctors can distinguish simple dry eye from eye allergy because of a distinctive "cobblestone" pattern seen inside the eyelids in those with allergies. Contact lens wearers are particularly vulnerable to eye allergy.

Drops prescribed to treat allergic eyes contain antihistamines, decongestants, or cortisone. They reduce inflammation but treat only the symptom, not the source of the problem, and they can make dry eyes worse. Continual use of any of them can damage the eyes. To better control allergies at their source, have yourself tested so that you know which allergens to avoid most carefully. If you are most allergic to dust mite droppings, you can buy mite-proof pillow and bed casings, an air filtration system, and a top-quality vacuum cleaner. Getting rid of carpeting and extra dust-collecting objects is also important if you have a dust mite allergy. If you are allergic to pollens, keep your windows closed and use an air-conditioner during the allergy season. Know the hours during which the pollens and molds you are most sensitive to are heaviest in outdoor air. Stay indoors during those hours. Usually the worst times are between the hours of 5 and 10 A.M. If you do go out, wear wraparound sun goggles to keep out dust and pollen.

To control allergic reactions, try the bioflavonoid quercetin, 500 mg twice a day. It's a natural hista-

mine blocker, so it works much like those antihista-
mine drugs but without the side effects. Take it with
vitamin C, one of nature's most potent anti-inflammatory agents. We recommend that you take 2–3 g
(2,000–3,000 mg) of vitamin C daily anyway, but you
may want to try taking 1,000 mg four times a day if
you have allergies. Some companies make products
that combine quercetin with vitamin C. Echinacea,
an herb that fortifies the immune system, is available
in a tincture (liquid) form. This can be added to your
allergy control regimen.

IN SHORT . . .

1.  Choose sunglasses carefully. Make sure they cut out 100 percent of the sun's ultraviolet radiation. Remember that the label's claims may not be accurate.

2.  Eye drops are used daily by many people with eye problems, particularly those with glaucoma, dry eye, or eye allergies. It's important to use eye drops correctly. If you use artificial tears, find a brand that doesn't contain benzalkonium chloride or other harmful preservatives. Wash hands before putting in eye drops and keep the bottle in a place where it's least likely to become contaminated with bacteria. Refrigerated eye drops can be soothing to the eyes.

3.  Dry eyes can be caused by a variety of medications, by preservatives used in some eye drops, or by nutritional deficiencies. Try the following supplements for dry eyes:

    Omega-6 fatty acids from evening primrose, borage, or black currant seed oil

    Omega-3 fatty acids from fish

    Vitamin $B_6$ to improve utilization of essential fatty acids (50 mg)

Preservative-free vitamin A drops (VIVA Drops by Vision Pharmaceuticals)

Plenty of vitamin A and beta-carotene-rich foods in the diet

Vitamin C (1,000–4,000 mg a day in divided doses)

Clean water—lots of it

Glucosamine sulfate (500 mg twice a day)

4. Also try your best to avoid using medications or artificial sweeteners that dry the eyes out. Plugging the tear drains may be an effective way to remedy dry eyes that don't respond to nutritional changes.

5. Your first step in treating an eye allergy is to try to eliminate allergenic substances from the surroundings and from the diet. Vitamin C, quercetin (500 mg twice a day), and echinacea can be helpful in reducing inflammation that causes allergy symptoms.

# 15

# Coping with Vision Loss

Loss of vision can be emotionally devastating. For older people, it often means loss of independence. Check writing, grocery shopping, the use of a computer, reading, watching television, and other daily tasks and recreations that once were so easy become difficult or impossible. It's not unusual for the loss of vision to bring about bouts of deep depression. Having to depend upon others makes many still strong, vital people with low vision (due to macular degeneration, glaucoma, cataracts, diabetic eye disease, or retinitis pigmentosa) feel much more helpless than they actually are.

Thanks to modern technology, people with low vision can make the most of their remaining sight. There are dozens of gadgets to choose from that will make your life as a partially sighted person much easier. You don't have to give up the activities you love. You can remain in charge of your own finances and read those tiny labels in the grocery store.

For those who are totally blind, there are many options as well. Because most of the people who will benefit from this book don't fall into this category, this chapter will focus on how to enhance remaining sight. If you would like information or resources on aids for the totally blind, contact the American Foundation for the Blind at (800) 829-0500.

## About Low-Vision Aids

There are three categories used to classify low-vision aids:

**1. Optical aids:** These are used to control focus and clarify or magnify images. They include magnifying glasses, spectacles, clip-on jewelers' loupes (these single-eye magnifiers can be attached to glasses for fine, detailed work such as embrodiery), absorptive lenses, visual aids that are worn on the head (to allow comfortable distance viewing of television, movies, or plays), and telescopes.

**2. Nonoptical aids and approach magnification:** These are steps you can take to control illumination and contrast to improve vision. Moving closer to an object, using brighter lights, and the use of reading and typing stands, filters, pinholes, tints, large print, visors, side shields, and guides to help with handwriting and check writing fall into this category.

**3. Electronic aids:** Closed-circuit television, where a book is magnified on your TV screen, is an example. In this age of computers, there are countless programs and hardware you can install to make your computer a useful and versatile tool for coping with vision loss.

In this chapter we will give you some general information about low-vision aids. In Appendix II is a listing of some of the organizations that can help you to make the most of your remaining vision. It's important that you sit down with your ophthalmologist or an experienced low-vision specialist to discuss your options. He or she will try to understand your needs and will help you to obtain the devices best suited to your lifestyle. Ask your eye doctor to recommend a low-vision consultant in your area.

## Learning to Use Peripheral Vision When You Have Macular Degeneration

For those with macular degeneration, mastery of a technique called *eccentric viewing* gives you full use of remaining vision. Since the blind spot is always at the very center of your visual field, you can look slightly off center. This allows you to look around the blind spot to better see the television, food on your plate, or faces you might otherwise not recognize. Try making a habit of looking at one corner of the TV screen. It takes some practice, and you will need to experiment to find your ideal off-center focus. You'll be surprised at how much you can see once you've mastered this technique.

## Magnifiers

There are many kinds of magnifiers for you to choose from. For hands-free viewing, you can use magnifiers that clamp onto the edge of your desk. They usually have flexible necks that allow you to move the glass around as needed. There are other models you can hang around your neck or that are worn on a headband. Large magnifiers can be mounted on four legs and placed over a book.

Hand-held magnifying glasses, often with small lights mounted in the frame, can be found in many sizes and shapes to fit in pocket or purse. You usually can find these at the drugstore. Magnifiers with high-powered halogen lights are especially good for those with poor dim-light vision. Aspheric magnifiers help eliminate irregularities in images so that you can have powerful magnification while having a large field of view.

Bar readers are long and slender, designed for magnification of a single line of text on a page. Page viewers allow you to magnify most of a page for ease in reading maps or text. Lighted fold-up magnifiers are great for reading labels or coupons at the market. Jewelers' loupes—used by jewelers and watchmakers for very fine work—can be held to the eye or mounted on glasses. If you love to build models, embroider, or do other handiwork, loupes are indispensable. (You can buy them at camera shops.) Magnifying mirrors allow you to apply makeup, shave, and groom with a clear view.

For distance viewing, you can use focusable

binocular glasses. Wearing them on a headband is comfortable for long viewing periods at movies or shows. A focusable monocular held up to the eye is good for intermittent distance viewing.

## Nonoptical Aids and Approach Magnification

Bring plenty of light into your home. Adjustable halogen lamps with high-wattage bulbs can be mounted above work to create a wide pool of light. Special lamps and filters can improve contrast. Carry a halogen-light pocket magnifier with you to see better in dim restaurants and shops.

Large-print reading materials are widely available; check Appendix II.

Books on tape can be bought or borrowed from the library. Interlibrary loan of these materials is available, and you can listen to novels, nonfiction, or even textbooks.

Handwriting guides allow you to write letters and checks neatly.

## Electronic Aids

For comfortable low-vision reading, you can use a closed-circuit TV system. These can be used with any television set. The document you're reading is placed beneath a small camera, which brings the text onto your TV screen. You can enlarge it as much as you want, and some systems allow you to read either dark letters on light background or white on dark (the latter can reduce glare). This tool can be used for writing as well. A movable platform allows you to move reading or writing material in any direction. You'll be able to pay your own bills, read your own mail, and enjoy reading books. A company called Okay Vision-Aide Corporation sells many different closed-circuit TV models at reasonable prices, and they give you plenty of instruction and support when you use their products. They can be reached at (800) 325-4488.

Visionics Corporation makes special binoculars, worn on the head, that allow you to program in your eyeglass prescription so that you don't need to wear glasses while using them. You can use a complex set of controls to zoom in on objects across the room or to see up close. It's like wearing a video camera on your head. It's a new gadget, very bulky and not easy to use, but if you'd like more information you can call (800) 684-7834.

## Computer Applications

Many older folks are intimidated by computers. Five-year-olds are already "surfing the Net," but those of us accustomed to typewriters and libraries have trouble adjusting to the world of word processing and CD-ROMs. However, it's truly astonishing what you can do with the right computer system, and for partially sighted people it can be a liberating tool.

To enlarge text on the screen, you can use the "zoom" feature included in many word-processing programs. You also can buy large magnifying screens to put over your computer screen. Programs like inLarge, from Berkeley Access (a division of Berkeley Systems, Inc., which specializes in low-vision computer applications), allow you to enlarge text or graphics from two to sixteen times. Berkeley Systems also makes a terrific, inexpensive text-to-voice translator for the Macintosh computer, as well as portable video reading systems with light headsets that you quickly can connect to any TV or monitor.

Text-to-voice translator programs or speech synthesizers can be used with your computer. Having text read to you as you read it yourself will allow you to read quickly and with great accuracy. A programmer named John F. Adams has invented a system he calls "Proportional Reading," which allows the reader to display one sentence or even one word at a time on the screen as a voice reads it. This could be very useful for those with macular degeneration because the eyes don't have to move along the page. Your focus could remain on one corner of the screen, and you comfortably could use your peripheral vision. His E-mail address is *proread@tiac.net*. If you want to read materials other than those that can be bought on disc or CD-ROM, you can use a scanner that brings text from the page onto your screen.

A company called Universal Low Vision Aids sells and rents closed-circuit TVs as well as computer hardware and software. Many of the manufacturers I've mentioned sell their products through this company. Universal Low Vision Aids also carries computer programs that allow you to

- fill out preprinted forms using your computer; and
- use any video monitor or TV as a monitor for your computer. (Imagine—a big-screen TV as a computer monitor!)

Training and technical support is provided with their products. Call them at (614) 486-0098 to find out more.

Don't let yourself be intimidated by computers. All the help you need is available from representatives of the company whose computer you buy. If you don't have a computer yet, it's a good idea to sit down with a low-vision-aids consultant before shopping for one. Make sure you have the best model with all the needed hardware so that you can use these special programs.

**IN SHORT . . .**

1. If you have lost much of your vision, there are tools and gadgets in abundance that can help you to maintain your independence and your quality of life.

2. Sit down with your ophthalmologist or a low-vision-aids consultant to decide which low-vision aids will work the best for you.

3. Take advantage of the many organizations dedicated to improving the lives of partially sighted people. If there are any support groups in your area, try to attend meetings. Having the support of others with similar problems will improve your sense of well-being dramatically and diminish frustrations.

# Appendix I:

# A Summary of Nutritional Prescriptions for Eye Disease

## Your Daily Multivitamin Should Include . . .

Beta-carotene/carotenoids: 10,000–15,000 IU
Vitamin A: 5,000–10,000 IU
The B Vitamins:
    Thiamine ($B_1$): 25–50 mg
    Riboflavin ($B_2$): 25–100 mg
    Niacin ($B_3$): 50–100 mg
    Pantothenic acid ($B_5$): 50–100 mg
    Pyridoxine ($B_6$): 50–100 mg
    Vitamin $B_{12}$: 1,000–2,000 micrograms (mcg)
    Biotin: 100–300 mcg
    Choline: 50–100 mg
    Folic acid (folate or folacin): 400–800 mcg
    Inositol: 150–300 mg
Calcium: 300–500 mg for men; 600–1,200 mg for women

Vitamin D: 100–400 IU
Vitamin C: 2,000–10,000 mg (2–10 g)
Vitamin E: 400–800 IU
Boron: 1–5 mg
Chromium: 200–400 mcg, as chromium picolinate
Copper: 1–5 mg
Magnesium: 300–500 mg
Manganese: 10 mg
Selenium: 25–50 mcg
Vanadyl sulfate: 10–25 mcg
Zinc: 10–30 mg

The recommended amounts of nutrients in the following "nutritional prescriptions" are in addition to your daily multivitamin, unless specified otherwise.

## Daily Nutritional Prescription for Macular Degeneration

Vitamin C and bioflavonoids: at least 2,000 mg of vitamin C, and 200–400 mg of bioflavonoids
Beta-carotene: 15,000–25,000 IU
Vitamin A: 10,000–25,000 IU, for three months
Lutein and zeaxanthin: 6–10 mg
Magnesium: 300–500 mg, at bedtime
Fish Oils: Follow the directions on the container.
Vitamin E: 800 IU (total)
Selenium: at least 200 mcg
N-acetyl cysteine (NAC): 500 mg, 2–3 times
Taurine: 500–1,000 mg, between meals
Garlic: about 1,000 mg of the odorless capsules
Zinc: 15–30 mg, if your multivitamin is low in zinc

Coenzyme Q10: 30–200 mg
Hydrochloric acid: 250 mg, with meals, if needed

## Daily Nutritional Prescription
## for Glaucoma

Vitamin C: 1,000 mg
Vitamin E: as recommended in your multivitamin
Beta-carotene: 25,000 IU
Carotenoids: Use a mixed carotenoid supplement at different times from your food ingestion of beta-carotene (see page 96).
Vitamin A: 5,000–10,000 IU
Quercetin: 1,000–3,000 mg
Rutin: 1,000–3,000 mg
Magnesium: 250–400 mg, at bedtime
Vitamin B complex: as recommended in your multivitamin
Vitamin $B_{12}$: 1,000–2,000 mcg (Since it is not well absorbed when taken orally, take it sublingually—under the tongue—or use a nasal spray or gel.)
Zinc: as recommended in your multivitamin
Coenzyme Q10: 90–200 mg (Use with ginger root capsules for added effect if you have low-pressure glaucoma; this will increase your heart's pumping capacity.)
Carnitine: 500 mg, to strengthen the heart's pumping power
Omega-3 oils found in fish (see page 98). (DHA, a component of omega-3 oils, is a component of the optic nerve lining.)

Garlic: 1 raw clove, with food; or 1,000 mg of the odorless capsules

Coleus (forskolin): 200–400 mg

Chromium: 200–600 mg if you are using beta-blocker eye drops, to help boost HDL cholesterol

## Daily Nutritional Prescription for Cataracts

Vitamin E: as recommended in your multivitamin

Vitamin C: 1,000–2,000 mg

Beta-carotene: 10,000–25,000 IU

Vitamin A: 5,000–10,000 IU

Zinc: 15–30 mg (total for the day)

N-acetyl cysteine (NAC): 500 mg, 2–3 times between meals

Rutin (a bioflavonoid): 250 mg

Quercetin (another bioflavonoid): 1,000–3,000 mg

Chromium: 200 mcg

Riboflavin: 50 mg (If you need to add to your multivitamin, do so.)

Coenzyme Q10: 30–90 mg

Curcumin (turmeric): liberally as a spice, or taken as a supplement according to directions on the bottle

## Daily Nutritional Prescription for Diabetic Eye Disease

Vitamin C: 1,000 mg (This may alter the color of urine strips.)

B vitamins: as recommended in your multivitamin

Vitamin E: as recommended in your multivitamin

Beta-carotene: as recommended in your multivitamin

Quercetin: 500–1,000 mg

Chromium: 100–200 mcg

Vanadyl Sulfate: 10–20 mg

Magnesium: 400 mg, at bedtime

N-acetyl cysteine: 500 mg, 2–3 times between meals

Omega-3 oils from cold-water fish (see page 98)

Garlic: 1 raw clove, with food; or 1,000 mg of the
odorless capsules

Zinc: as recommended in your multivitamin

Carnitine: 500 mg

Alpha lipoic acid: 500 mg in divided doses (Use caution; it may cause your blood sugar to dip precipitously.)

## Daily Nutritional Prescription for Retinitis Pigmentosa

Vitamin E: as recommended in your multivitamin

Vitamin C and bioflavonoids: 1,000–2,000 mg and
250–400 mg, respectively

Beta-carotene: as recommended in your multivitamin

(Take all of the above antioxidants together, so they
can re-energize one another as they work.)

Lutein/zeaxanthin: 6–12 mg, at different times from
your food ingestion of beta-carotene

Zinc: as recommended in your multivitamin

B vitamins: as recommended in your multivitamin

N-acetyl cysteine (NAC): 500 mg, 2–3 times between meals

Quercetin (another bioflavonoid): 500–1,500 mg

Bilberry, grapeseed, and cranberry extracts: (These are other good sources of bioflavonoids, which help vitamin C to strengthen capillaries in the eyes.) Follow dosage instructions on the container.

Coenzyme Q10: 30–200 mg

Magnesium: 300–400 mg

Carnitine: 300–1,500 mg

Cayenne pepper capsules: 1–2 capsules with meals to help relieve headaches

Ginkgo biloba: 120–360 mg

Alpha lipoic acid: 100–300 mg

Taurine: 1,000 mg (taken with 800 IU vitamin E, divided into 2 doses) if you have the autosomal dominant form of RP, or if you have Usher's syndrome

## Daily Nutritional Prescription for Clear, Strong Blood Vessels

Vitamin C: as recommended in your multivitamin, and up to 10,000 mg (10 g) if needed

Vitamin E: as recommended in your multivitamin

Magnesium: as recommended in your multivitamin

Folic acid: as recommended in your multivitamin

Vitamin $B_6$: as recommended in your multivitamin

Vitamin $B_3$ (niacin) in the form of inositol hexanicotinate: 100 mg

Vitamin B$_{12}$: 1,000–2,000 mcg sublingually or intranasally

N-acetyl cysteine (NAC): 500 mg, 2–3 times

Lysine: 300–500 mg, 3 times

Proline: 300–500 mg, 3 times

CoQ10: 30–90 mg, in the liquid oil form

Carnitine: 100–150 mg

Betaine hydrochloride: a 300-mg tablet, increasing the amount if needed, with meals to improve digestion and absorption of B vitamins

# Appendix II:

# Resources

## For More Information on Intravenous Nutrients

Call or write the American College for Advancement in Medicine, listed below under "Chelation Information,"

or

Order *Nutritional Therapy in Medical Practice*, by Alan R. Gaby, M.D., and Jonathan Wright, M.D., by writing Wright/Gaby Seminars, 515 W. Harrison Street, Suite 200, Kent, WA 98032, or calling (206) 854-4900, ext. 166.

## Chelation Information and Referrals to Alternative Health Care Professionals

American College for Advancement in Medicine (ACAM)
P.O. Box 3427
Laguna Hills, CA 92654
(800) 532-3688
In California: (714) 583-7666

## Mail Order Vitamins

The Vitamin Shoppe, Call 1-800-223-1216 to order a catalog.

Life Extension Vitamins 1-800-544-4440

# Organizations for the Partially Sighted and Blind

## Support, Information, and Low-Vision Aids

National Association for the Visually Handicapped
22 W. 21st Street
New York, NY 10010
(212) 889-3141
Fax: (212) 727-2931

Provides counseling in the testing, purchase, and use of low-vision aids and special illumination for the low-vision reader. A catalog is available. The NAVH also offers a large-print lending library by mail, with over five thousand titles to choose from. They put together a newsletter and offer educational materials on eye diseases and emotional support for those individuals and their families who suffer from them.

Council of Citizens with Low Vision International (CCLVI)
5707 Brockton Drive, #302
Indianapolis, IN 46220-5481
(800) 733-2258
(317) 254-1332
Fax: (317) 251-6599

State and regional chapters offer newsletter and low-vision resources.

Glaucoma Support Network
Glaucoma Research Foundation
490 Post Street
San Francisco, CA 94102
(800) 826-6693
(415) 986-3162
E-mail: glaucoma@itsa.ucsf.edu

A national telephone network for glaucoma patients and their families. Support and encouragement from volunteers help patients cope with vision loss from glaucoma. The Glaucoma Research Foundation sponsors and conducts research, provides patient education and support services, publishes *Gleams* (a quarterly newsletter) and a patient guide about treatments, therapies, and coping with glaucoma.

Lighthouse National Center for Vision and Aging
111 E. 59th Street
New York, NY 10022
(800) 334-5497
(212) 821-9713

Clearinghouse of support groups for visually impaired older people. Publishes a directory of self-help and mutual-aid support groups and a newsletter. The **Lighthouse Center for Education,** another branch of this organization, provides information, resources, education, and professionally prepared multimedia and print materials for community education lectures. Technical consultations and catalog available.

The Lighthouse, Inc.
Consumer Products
36-02 Northern Boulevard
Long Island City, NY 11101
(800) 829-0500
(718) 937-6959

Publishes a catalog of nonoptical devices and products for daily living.

Independent Living Aids, Inc.
27 E. Mall
Plainview, NY 11803
(800) 537-2118
(516) 752-8080
Fax: (516) 752-3135

Publishes a catalog of low-vision devices for daily living.

Macular Degeneration Awareness
Education Support Group Against All Odds, Inc.
Contact: Morton Bond
700 S. Hollybrook Drive #210
Pembroke Pines, FL 33025
(305) 431-3111

Nonprofit organization providing awareness, education, and support.

Macular Degeneration Foundation Education, Inc.
P.O. Box 9752
San Jose, CA 95157-9752
(408) 260-1335
Fax: (408) 260-1336

E-mail: mdfeyes@aimnet.com
    eyesight@eyesight.com

Nonprofit corporation that provides a newsletter and other support services to the visually impaired.

National Diabetes Information Clearinghouse
1 Information Way
Bethseda, MD 20892-3560
(301) 654-3327

Provides publications on diabetes. Answers requests for specialized information, publishes quarterly bulletin, and maintains a database of diabetes educational materials.

The Foundation Fighting Blindness
Executive Plaza 1, Suite 800
11350 McCormick Road
Hunt Valley, MD 21031-1014
(888) 394-3937
(800) 683-5551
(410) 785-1414
(410) 785-9687
Fax: (410) 771-9470

Provides information for those with retinal degenerative diseases (such as macular degeneration and retinitis pigmentosa). Call one of the toll-free numbers for a listing of support groups in your area.

Independent Living Aids, Inc.
27 E. Mall
Plainview, NY 11803
(800) 537-2118

(516) 752-8080
(516) 752-3135

American Council of the Blind
1155 15th Street NW, Suite 720
Washington, DC 20005
(800) 424-8666 (weekdays 3–5:30 P.M. Eastern time)
(202) 467-5081
(800) 424-8666 (6 P.M. to midnight in Washington, DC)

National membership organization of the blind with state, local, and special-interest chapters; free monthly magazine in large print and Braille, on cassette and on disk.

National Federation of the Blind
1800 Johnson Street
Baltimore, MD 21230
(410) 659-9314

National organization with local chapters of partially sighted and blind members. Offers national magazine and literature in print and Braille, and on cassette. Maintains referral and job services.

## Large-Print Reading Materials

American Printing House for the Blind
1839 Frankfort Avenue
PO Box 6085
Louisville, KY 40206-0085
(800) 223-1839

(502) 895-2405
(502) 899-2274
E-mail: aph@iglou.com

Large-type textbooks, cookbooks, and dictionaries. Call for a free catalog and semi-annual newsletters in 14-point type.

Blindskills, Inc.
PO Box 5181
Salem, OR 97304-0181
(503) 581-4224
Fax: (503) 581-0178

Publishes quarterly magazine, *Dialogue*, in large print and Braille, or on tape.

Doubleday Large Print Home Library
Membership Services Center
6550 East 30th Street
PO Box 6325
Indianapolis, IN 46206
(317) 541-8920

Large-print and cassette editions of best-sellers.

G. K. Hall and Company/Thorndike Press
PO Box 159
Thorndike, ME 04986
(800) 223-6121
(207) 948-2962
Fax: (800) 558-4676 (toll-free)

Direct sale of large-print books.

John Milton Society for the Blind
475 Riverside Drive, Room 455
New York, NY 10115
(212) 870-3336
Fax: (212) 870-3229

Provides free large-type directory of resources and free Christian literature in large type and Braille, and on cassette.

Library of Congress
National Library Services for the Blind and Physically Handicapped
1291 Taylor Street, NW
Washington, DC 20542
(800) 424-8567
(202) 707-5100
(202) 707-0744
Fax: (202) 707-0712

Administers a national library service that provides Braille and recorded books and magazines on free loan to those who can't read standard print due to visual or physical disability.

*New York Times*/Large Print Weekly
229 W. 43rd Street
New York, NY 10036
(800) 631-2580 for large-type weekly subscriptions
(212) 556-1734 (main office)

Offers large-print *New York Times* subscriptions for home or business delivery.

*Reader's Digest*/Large Type Edition
PO Box 241

Mount Morris, IL 61054
(800) 877-5293
(815) 734-6963

Offers subscriptions to large-print *Reader's Digest*.
Condensed books, the Great Biographies series, and
the Bible are also available in large print.

The World at Large, Inc.
1689 46th Street
Brooklyn, NY 11204
(800) 285-2743
(718) 972-4000
Fax: (718) 972-9400

Biweekly large-print newspaper that prints articles
from magazines such as *U.S. News and World Report*,
*Time*, and the *Christian Science Monitor*.

Ulverscroft Large Print (USA), Inc.
PO Box 1230
West Seneca, NY 14224-1230
(800) 955-9659
(716) 674-4270
(716) 674-4195

Direct sale of large-print books.

## Recorded Reading Materials

American Printing House for the Blind
1839 Frankfort Avenue
PO Box 6085
Louisville, KY 40206-0085
(800) 223-1839

(502) 895-2405
Fax: (502) 899-2274
E-mail: aph@iglou.com

Provides free subscriptions to *Newsweek* and other magazines on cassette, *Reader's Digest* on cassette or in Braille, and a catalog on cassette listing educational resources.

Associated Services for the Blind
919 Walnut Street
Philadelphia, PA 19107
(800) 876-5456 (toll-free retail outlet offering products for the visually impaired, 10 A.M.–4 P.M. Eastern time)
(215) 627-0600
Fax: (215) 627-0692

Produces large-print, cassette, and Braille materials for the visually impaired in the business community.

Books on Tape, Inc.
PO Box 7900
Newport Beach, CA 92658-7900
(800) 626-3333

Rentals of books on tape from classics to best-sellers.

Braille Circulating Library
2700 Stuart Avenue
Richmond, VA 23220-3305
(804) 359-3743
Fax: (804) 359-4777

Books on cassette and in Braille, as well as large-print materials.

Choice Magazine Listening
85 Channel Drive
Port Washington, NY 11050-2216
(516) 883-8280
Fax: (516) 944-6849

Selected unabridged articles on cassette bimonthly, free of charge, from popular print magazines.

Christian Record Services, Inc.
4444 S. 52nd Street
PO Box 6097
Lincoln, NE 68506
(402) 488-0981
Fax: (402) 488-7582
    (402) 488-1902

Provides free Christian publications and programs for the visually or hearing impaired. Magazines in large print and Braille, or on cassette, a lending library, a Bible correspondence school, and other services are available.

Jewish Braille Institute of America, Inc.
110 E. 30th Street
New York, NY 10016
(212) 889-2525

Large-print, Braille, and talking books.

Jewish Guild for the Blind
15 W. 65th Street
New York, NY 10023
(212) 769-6200

Provides a radio reading service and books on tape. Offers comprehensive low-vision evaluations and services.

Recording for the Blind and Dyslexic
The Anne T. MacDonald Center
20 Roszel Road
Princeton, NJ 08540
(800) 221-4792
(609) 452-0606

Provides free educational and professional materials on tape to help those with reading problems pursue their chosen occupations. Direct sale of books on computer disk and specially adapted players and recorders.

Xavier Society for the Blind
154 E. 23rd Street
New York, NY 10010
(800) 637-9193
(212) 473-7800
Fax: (212) 473-7801

Inspirational and religious materials in large-print, tape, and Braille formats. Catholic periodicals, Bible program, lending library, and religion textbooks are also available.

## General Information and Referral Services

American Academy of Ophthalmology
Public Information Program
PO Box 7424
San Francisco, CA 94120-7424

(415) 561-8500
E-mail: ips@aao.org

Brochures and eye fact sheets on eye conditions and visual impairment.

American Foundation for the Blind
11 Penn Plaza, Suite 300
New York, NY 10001
(800) 232-5463
(212) 502-7600
(212) 620-2158
(212) 620-2147 (NY residents)

Offers consultation services to eye-care, rehabilitation, and education professionals, serves as a national clearinghouse for information about blindness, publishes "Directory of Agencies Serving the Visually Handicapped," and maintains regional offices throughout the United States.

National Eye Institute
Information Office
Building 31, Room 6A32
31 Center Drive MSC 2510
Bethesda, MD 20892-2510
(301) 496-5248

Provides publications on eye diseases and information on current eye research.

Prevent Blindness America (formerly National Society to Prevent Blindness)
500 E. Remington Road
Schaumburg, IL 60173

(800) 331-2020
(708) 843-2020

Publishes a variety of information on vision, eye health, and safety. Provides information on eye research and some community services.

Resources for Rehabilitation
33 Bedford Street, Suite 19A
Lexington, MA 02173
(617) 862-6455
Fax: (617) 861-7517

Publishes large-print directories such as *Living with Low Vision: A Resource Guide for People with Sight Loss* and *Resources for Elders with Disabilities*, as well as large-print resource lists.

VISION Foundation, Inc.
818 Mt. Auburn Street
Watertown, MA 02172
(800) 852-3029
(617) 926-4232
Fax: (617) 926-1412

Publishes the *VISION Resource List*, available in large print or cassette.

Visions/Services for the Blind and Visually Impaired
120 Wall Street, 16th Floor
New York, NY 10005-3904
(212) 425-2255
Fax: (212) 425-7114

Offers free services to anyone over age fifty-five with

vision problems, including self-help study kits, rehabilitation training in the home, and a year-round vacation camp for blind adults and their families.

## Recommended Reading

### General Nutrition and Wellness

Batmanghelidj, F., M.D. *Your Body's Many Cries for Water*. Falls Church, Va.: Global Health Solutions, Inc., 1995.

Bland, John H., M.D. *Live Long, Die Fast*. Minneapolis: Fairview Press, 1997.

Blaylock, Russell. *Excitotoxins: The Taste That Kills*. Sante Fe, N.M.: Health Press, 1994.

D'Adamo, Peter, N.D. *Eat Right 4 Your Type*. New York: Putnam, 1996.

Fallon, Sally. *Nourishing Traditions*. San Diego: ProMotion Publishing, 1995.

Golan, Ralph, M.D. *Optimal Wellness*. New York: Ballantine Books, 1995.

Jahnke, Roger. *The Healer Within*. San Francisco: HarperCollins, 1997.

Mindell, Earl, R.Ph., Ph.D., and Virginia Hopkins. *Dr. Earl Mindell's What You Should Know About . . . Series*. New Canaan, Conn.: Keats Publishing, 1996.

Morton, Mary and Michael. *Five Steps to Selecting the Best Alternative Medicine*. Novato, Calif.: New World Library, 1996.

Pauling, Linus. *How To Live Longer and Feel Better*. New York: Avon Books, 1987.

———. *Vitamin C and the Common Cold*. Tampa Bay, Fla.: Buccanneer Books, Inc., 1995.

Pizzorno, Joseph N. *Total Wellness*, Rocklin, Calif: Prima Publishing, 1996.

Robbins, John. *Reclaiming Our Health*. Tiburon, Calif.: H. J. Kramer, 1996.

Sears, Barry. *The Zone*. New York: HarperCollins, 1996.

Todd, Gary Price, M.D. *Nutrition, Health, and Disease*. West Chester, Pa.: Whitford Press, 1985.

## Detoxifying

Casdorph, R. H., M.D., and Morton Walker, M.D. *Toxic Metal Syndrome: How Metal Poisonings Can Affect Your Brain*. Garden City, N.Y.: Avery Publishing Group, 1995.

Golan, Ralph, M.D. *Optimal Wellness*. New York: Ballantine Books, 1995.

Walker, Morton, M.D. *The Chelation Way*. Garden City, N.Y.: Avery Publishing Group, 1990.

## Hormone Balance And Xenobiotics:

Barnes, Broda. *Hypothyroidism: The Unsuspected Illness*. New York: Harper and Row, 1976.

Colburn, Theo. *Our Stolen Future: Are We Threatening Our Fertility, Intelligence and Survival?* New York: Plume Books, 1997.

Khalsa, Dharma Singh, M.D. *Brain Longevity*. New York: Warner Books, 1997.

Klatz, Ronald, and Robert Goldman. *Stopping the Clock*. New York: Bantam Books, 1996.

Klatz, Ronald, with Carol Kahn. *Grow Young with HGH*. New York: HarperCollins, 1997.

Lee, John R., M.D., and Virginia Hopkins. *What Your Doctor May Not Tell You about Menopause: The Breakthrough Book on Natural Progesterone*. New York: Warner Books, 1996.

Sahelian, Ray. *Melatonin: Nature's Sleeping Pill*. Garden City, N.Y.: Avery Publishing, 1995.

———*DHEA: A Practical Guide*. Garden City, N.Y.: Avery Publishing, 1996.

## Staying Healthy in a Toxic World

Hunter, Linda Mason. *The Healthy Home: An Attic-to-Basement Guide to Toxin-Free Living*. New York: Pocket Books, 1990.

Steinman, David, and Michael Wisner. *Living Healthy in a Toxic World*. New York: The Berkley Publishing Group, 1996.


## Drugs

Breggin, Peter. *Talking Back to Prozac*. New York: St. Martin's Press, 1994.

Mindell, Earl, and Virginia Hopkins. *Prescription Alternatives*. New Canaan, Conn.: Keats Publishing, 1998.

# Appendix III:

# References

## Chapter 2: How Your Eyes Work

Gottsch J, et al. "Light-induced deposits in Bruch's membrane of protoporphyric mice." *Archives of Ophthalmology* 111(1):126–9, 1993 Jan.

Rozanowska M, et al. "Blue light–induced reactivity of retinal age pigment: In vitro generation of oxygen-reactive species." *Journal of Biological Chemistry* 270(32):18825–30, 1995 Aug 11.

## Chapter 3: The Nutritional Care and Feeding of Your Eyes

Almendingen K, et al. "Effects of partially hydrogenated fish oil, partially hydrogenated soybean oil, and butter on hemostatic variables in men." *Atherosclerosis, Thrombosis, and Vascular Biology* 16:373–80, 1996.

Benzer W, et al. "Effects of intravenous magnesium chloride reverses left ventricular end-diastolic pressure in coronary artery disease." *American Journal of Cardiology* 77:638–40, 1996 Mar.15.

Brichard S, Henquin J. "The role of vanadium in the management of diabetes." *Trends in Pharmacological Sciences* 16(8):265–70, 1995 Aug.

Bunker VW. "The role of nutrition in osteoporosis." *British Journal of Biomedical Science* 51(3):228–40, 1994 Sep.

Hamel F, Duckworth W. "The relationship between insulin and vanadium metabolism in insulin target tissues." *Molecular & Cellular Biochemistry* 153(1–2):95–102, 1995 Dec. 6–20.

Jacob RA, Burri BJ. "Oxidative damage and defense." *American Journal of Clinical Nutrition.* 63(6):985S–90S, 1996 Jun.

Jain S, ct al. "The effect of modest vitamin E supplementation on lipid peroxidation products and other cardiovascular risk factors in diabetic patients." *Lipids* 31(Suppl):S87–90, 1996 Mar.

Jha P, et al. "The antioxidant vitamins and cardiovascular disease: A critical review of epidemiologic and clinical trial data." *Annals of Internal Medicine* 123(11):860–72, 1995 Dec 1.

Julius M, et al. "Glutathione and morbidity in a community-based sample of elderly." *Journal of Clinical Epidemiology* 47(9):1021–6, 1994 Sep.

Keys A. "Coronary heart disease in seven countries." *Circulation* 41(4, 1 Suppl), 1970.

Mares-Perlman JA, et al. "Association of zinc and antioxidant nutrients with age-related maculopathy." *Archives of Ophthalmogy* 114(8):991–7, 1996 Aug.

Mo J, et al. "A new hypothesis about the relationship between free radical reactions and hemorheological properties in vivo." *Medical Hypotheses* 41(6):516–20, 1993 Dec.

Nastou H, et al. "Prophylactic effects of intravenous magnesium on hypertensive emergencies after cataract surgery: A new contribution to the pharmacological use of magnesium in anaesthesiology." *Magnesium Research* 8(3):271–6, 1995 Sep.

O'Keefe JH Jr, et al. "Insights into the pathogenesis and prevention of coronary artery disease." *Mayo Clinic Proceedings* 70(1):69–79, 1995 Jan.

Oliver MF. "Doubts about preventing coronary heart disease: Multiple interventions in middle-aged men may do more harm than good." *British Medical Journal* 304:593–4, 1992 Feb 15.

Snodderly DM. "Evidence for protection against ARMD by carotenoids and antioxidant vitamins." *American Journal of Clinical Nutrition* 62(6Suppl):1448S–61S, 1995 Dec.

Thomas SR. "Coantioxidants make alpha-tocopherol an efficient antioxidant for LDL." *American Journal of Clinical Nutrition* 62(6Suppl):1357S–64S, 1995 Dec.

Uay-Dagach R, Valenzuela A. "Marine oils as a source of omega-3 fatty acids in the diet: How to optimize the health benefits." *Progress in Food and Nutrition Science* 16(3):199–243, 1992.

Wynder EL. "Identification of women at high risk for breast cancer." *Cancer* 24:1235, 1969.

## Chapter 4: Preventing and Healing Macular Degeneration

Albert D MD, Jacobeic F MD D Sc(Med), Robinson N AB. *Principles and Practice of Ophthalmology: Basic Sciences*. Philadelphia: WB Saunders, 1994: 1266, 1272.

Bergink G, et al. "Radiation therapy for subfoveal choroidal neovascular membranes in age-related macular degeneration: A pilot study." *Graefes Archive for Clinical & Experimental Ophthalmology* 232(10):591–8, 1994 Oct.

Bernstein PS, Seddon JM. "Decision-making in the treatment of subfoveal neovascularization in age-related macular degeneration: An analysis from the patient's perspective." *Retina* 16(2):112–6, 1996.

Boulton M, et al. "Lipofuscin is a photoinducible free radical generator." *Journal of Photochemistry and Photobiology*. B-Biology 19(3):201–4, 1993 Aug.

Connor WE, et al. "Essential fatty acids: the importance of n-3 fatty acids in the retina and brain." *Nutrition Reviews* 50:21–9, 1992.

D'Amato RJ, et al. "Thalidomide is an inhibitor of angiogenesis." Proceedings of the National Academy of Sciences of the United States of America. 91(9):4082–5, 1994 Apr 26.

Dastgheib K, Bressler S, Green W. "Clinico-pathologic correlation of laser lesion expansion after treatment of choroidal neovascularization." *Retina* 13(4):345–52, 1993.

el Baba W, et al. "Massive hemorrhage complicating age-related macular degeneration: Clinicopathologic correlation and role of anticoagulants." *Ophthalmology* 93(12):1581–92, 1986 Dec.

Ferris FL. "Senile macular degeneration: review of epidemiologic features." *American Journal of Epidemiology* 118:132–50, 1983.

Finger P. "Radiation therapy for subretinal neovascularization." *Ophthalmology* 103(6):878–9, 1996 Jun.

Freund K, Yannuzzi L, Sorenson J. "Age-related macular degeneration and choroidal neovascularization." *American Journal of Ophthalmology* 115(6):786–91, 1993 Jun 15.

Goldberg J, et al. "Factors associated with age-related macular degeneration. An analysis of data from the first National Health and Nutrition Examination Survey." *American Journal of Epidemiology* 128(4):700–10, 1988 Oct.

Gutman M, et al. "Failure of thalidomide to inhibit tumor growth and angiogenesis in vivo." *Anticancer Research* 16(6B):3673–7, 1996 Nov–Dec.

Ip M, Gorin MB. "Recurrence of a choroidal neovascular membrane in a patient with punctate inner choroidopathy treated with daily doses of thalidomide." *American Journal of Ophthalmology* 122(4):594–5, 1996 Oct.

Johnson LE. "The emerging role of vitamins as antioxidants." *Archives of Family Medicine* 3(9):809–20, 1994, Sep.

Kaminski MS, et al. "Evaluation of dietary antioxidant levels and supplementation with ICAPS-Plus and Ocuvite." *Journal of the American Ophthalmology Association* 64(12):862–70, 1993 Dec.

Kirkpatrick JN, Dick AD, Forrester JV. "Clinical experience with interferon alfa-2a for exudative age-related macular degeneration." *British Journal of Ophthalmology* 77(12):766–70, 1993 Dec.

Klein R, et al. "Racial/ethnic differences in age-related maculopathy. Third National Health and Nutrition Examination Survey." *Ophthalmology* 102(3):371–81, 1995 Mar.

Leibowitz H, Krueger D, Mauder L. "The Framingham Eye Study Monograph." *Survey of Ophthalmology* 24(Suppl):1980.

Levy JG. "Photosensitizers in photodynamic therapy." *Seminars in Oncology* 21(6Suppl15):4–10, 1994 Dec.

McCarthy DM. "Mechanisms of mucosal injury and healing: the role of non-steroidal anti-inflammatory drugs." *Scandinavian Journal of Gastroenterology* 208(Suppl):24–9, 1995.

Munoz B, et al. "Blue light and risk of age-related macular degeneration." *Investigative Ophthalmology* 31:ARVO Abstracts, 1990 Mar 15.

Nordoy A. "Fish consumption and cardiovascular disease: A reappraisal." *Nutrition and Metabolism in Cardiovascular Disease* 6:103–9, 1996.

Richer S. "Atrophic armd—a nutrition responsive chronic disease." *Journal of the American Optomology Association* 67(1):6–10, 1996 Jan.

Richer S. "Multicenter Ophthalmic and nutritional age-related macular degeneration study—part 1: design, subjects and procedures." *Journal of the American Optomology Association* 67(1):12–29, 1996 Jan.

Richer SP. "Is there a prevention and treatment strategy for macular degeneration?" *Journal of the American Optomology Association* 64(12):838–50, 1993 Dec.

Sarma U, et al. "Nutrition and the epidemiology of cataract and age-related maculopathy." *European Journal of Clinical Nutrition* 48(1):1–8, 1994 Jan.

Seddon JM, et al. "Dietary carotenoids, vitamin A, C, and E and advanced age-related macular degeneration." *Journal of the American Medical Association* 272:1413–20, 1994.

Snodderly DM. "Evidence for protection against age-related macular degeneration by carotenoids and antioxidant vitamins." *American Journal of Clinical Nutrition* 62(6Suppl):1448S–61S, 1995 Dec.

Steiner M, et al. "A double-blind crossover study in moderately hypercholesterolemic men that compared the effect of aged garlic extract and placebo administration on blood lipids." *American Journal of Clinical Nutrition* 64:866–70, 1996.

Thoelen A, et al. "Treatment of choroidal neovascularization in age-related macular degeneration with interferon alfa-2a: a short term, nonrandomized pilot study." *German Journal of Ophthalmology* 4(3):137–43, 1995 May.

Traboulsi E, Jalkh A. "Retinal pigment epithelium tear as a cause of vitreous hemorrhage." *Annals of Ophthalmology* 17(4):228–30, 1985 Apr.

## Chapter 5: Preventing and Healing Glaucoma

Baudoin C, et al. "Expression of inflammatory membrane markers by conjunctival cells in chronically treated patients with glaucoma." *Ophthalmology* 101:454–60, 1994.

Caprioli J, Sears M. "Forskolin lowers intraocular pressure in rabbits, monkeys, and man." *Lancet* 1983:958–60, Apr 30.

Garbe E, et al. "Inhaled and nasal glucocorticoids and risk of ocular hypertension or open-angle glaucoma." *Journal of the American Medical Association* 277(9):722–7, 1997 Mar 5.

Hiett JA, and Dockter CA. "Topical carbonic anhydrase inhibitors: a new perspective in glaucoma therapy." *Optometry Clinics* 2(4):97–112, 1992.

Hugues FC, and LeJeunne C. "Systemic and local tolerability of ophthalmic drug formulations: An update." *Drug Safety* 8(5):365–80, 1993 May.

Jonas J, et al. "Parapapillary retinal diameter in normal and glaucomatous eyes." *Investigative Ophthalmology* 30:1599–1603, 1989.

Leydhecker W, Krieglstein GK. *Glaucoma Update II*. Berlin: Springer-Verlag, 1983:95–192.

Sakai T, Murata M, Amemiya T. "Effects of long-term treatment of glaucoma with vitamin $B_{12}$." *Glaucoma* 14:167–70, 1992.

Schweitzer D, et al. "Spectrometric investigation in ocular hypertension and early stages of primary open angle glaucoma and low tension glaucoma: Multisubstance analysis." *International Ophthalmology* 16:251–7, 1992.

Scott BT. "Topical carbonic anhydrase inhibitors: potential adjuvants to glaucoma therapy in the future." *Optometry & Vision Science* 71(5):332–8, 1994 May.

Serle JB. "Pharmacological advances in the treatment of glaucoma." *Drugs & Aging* 5(3):156–70, 1994 Sep.

Shingleton B, et al. "Long-term efficacy of argon laser trabeculoplasty: A 10-year follow-up study." *Ophthalmology* 100(9):1324–9, 1993 Sep.

Spaeth GL. *Ophthalmic Surgery: Principles and Practice*. Philadelphia: WB Saunders Company, 1990: 224–8.

White TC. "Aqueous shunt implant surgery for refractory glaucoma." *Journal of Ophthalmologic Nursing & Technology* 15(1):7–13, 1996 Jan–Feb.

Williams DE, et al. "Effects of timolol, betaxolol, and levobunolol on human tenon's fibroblasts in tissue culture." *Investigative Ophthalmology and Visual Sciences* 33:2233–41, 1992.

## Chapter 6: Preventing and Healing Cataracts

Awasthi S, et al. "Curcumin protects against 4-hydroxy-2-trans-nonenal-induced cataract formation in rat lenses." *American Journal of Clinical Nutrition* 64:761–6, 1996.

Chylack L Jr, Tung W, Harding R. "Sorbitol production in the lens: a means of counteracting glucose-derived osmotic stress." *Ophthalmic Research* 18(5):313–20, 1986.

Hankinson S, et al. "Nutrient intake and cataract extraction in women: A prospective study." *British Medical Journal* 305:335–9, 1992.

Jacques P, Chylack L. "Epidemiologic evidence of a role for the antioxidant vitamins and carotenoids in cataract prevention." *American Journal of Clinical Nutrition* 53(1Suppl):352S–5S, 1991 Jan.

Javitt C, et al. "Geographic variation in utilization of cataract surgery." *Medical Care* 33(1):90–105, 1995 Jan.

Jedziniak J, Arredondo M, Andley U. "Oxidative damage to human lens enzymes." *Current Eye Research* 6(2):345–50, 1987 Feb.

Malone J, Lewitt S, Cook W. "Nonosmotic diabetic cataracts." *Pediatric Research* 27(3):293–6, 1990 Mar.

Ordy JM, Brizzee KR, Johnson HA. "Cellular alterations in visual pathways and the limbic system: Implications for vision and short-term memory." *Aging and Human Visual Function*, R Sekuler, D Kline, K Dismukes, eds. New York: Alan R Liss, 1982:79–114.

Rathbun W, Bovis M. "Activity of glutathione peroxidase and glutathione reductase in the human lens related to age." *Current Eye Research* 5(5):381–5, 1986 May.

Robertson J, Donner A, Trevithick J. "A possible role for vitamins C and E in cataract prevention." *American Journal of Clinical Nutrition* 53(1Suppl):335S–45S, 1991 Jan.

Robertson J, Donner A, Trevithick J. "Vitamin E and risk of cataract in humans." *Annals of the New York Academy of Sciences* 570:372–82, 1989.

Spaeth GL, ed. *Ophthalmic Surgery: Principles and Practice*. Philadelphia: WB Saunders, 1990: 162–3.

Sperduto R, et al. "The Linxian cataract studies: Two nutrition intervention trials." *Archives of Ophthalmology* 111(9):1246–53, 1993 Sep.

Varma S. "Scientific basis for medical therapy of cataracts by antioxidants." *American Journal of Clinical Nutrition* 53(1Suppl):335S–45S, 1991 Jan.

## Chapter 7: Preventing and Healing Diabetic Eye Disease

Barnard J, et al. "Response of non-insulin-dependent diabetic patients to an intensive program of diet and exercise." *Diabetes Care* 5:370–4, 1982 Jul–Aug.

Barnard J, et al. "Role of diet and exercise in the management of hyperinsulinemia and associated atherosclerotic risk factors." *American Journal of Cardiology* 69:440–4, 1992.

Cameron N, Cotter M. "Neurovascular effects of L-carnitine treatment in diabetic rats." *European Journal of Pharmacology* 319:239–44, 1997.

Challem J. "Antioxidants might ease diabetic complications." *Medical Tribune* 1996 Dec 12:18.

Chew EY, et al. "Effects of aspirin on vitreous/pre-retinal hemorrhage in patients with diabetes mellitus: Early Treatment Diabetic Retinopathy Study report no. 20." *Archives of Ophthalmology* 113(1):52–5, 1995 Jan.

Flynn HW Jr, et al. "Pars plana vitrectomy in the Early Treatment Diabetic Retinopathy Study, EDTRS report no. 17. The Early Treatment Diabetic Retinopathy Study Research Group." *Ophthalmology* 99(9):1351–7, 1992 Sep.

Jacob S, et al. "The antioxidant alpha-lipoic acid enhances insulin-stimulated glucose metabolism in insulin-resistant rat skeletal muscle." *Diabetes* 45(8):1024–9, 1996 Aug.

Kilic F, et al. "Modelling cortical caractogenesis 17: in vitro effect of a lipoic acid on glucose-induced lens membrane damage, a model of diabetic cataractogenesis." *Biochemistry & Molecular Biology International* 37(2):361–70, 1995 Oct.

Kowluru R, et al. "Abnormalities of retinal metabolism in diabetes or experimental galactosemia, III: Effects of antioxidants." *Diabetes* 45:1233–7, 1996.

Lovejoy J, DiGirolamo M. "Habitual dietary intake and insulin sensitivity in lean and obese adults." *American Journal of Clinical Nutrition* 55:1174–9, 1992.

Rubin R. "A tighter rein on diabetes." *US News & World Report*, 1993 June 28: 68.

Tuominen J, et al. "Exercise increases insulin clearance in healthy man and insulin dependent diabetes mellitus patients." *Clinical Physiology* 17:19–30, 1997.

Ziegler D, et al. "Treatment of symptomatic diabetic peripheral neuropathy with the anti-oxidant alpha-lipoic acid. A 3-week multicentre randomized controlled trial (ALADIN study)." *Diabetologica* 38(12):1425–33, 1995 Dec.

## Chapter 8: Preventing and Healing Retinitis Pigmentosa

Vingolo EM, et al. "Does hyperbaric oxygen (HBO) delivery rescue retinal photoreceptors in retinitis pigmentosa?" *Investigative Ophthalmology* 38: ARVO Abstracts, 1997.

## Chapter 9: There Is No Good Nutrition without Good Digestion

Fallon, Sally. *Nourishing Traditions*. San Diego, Calif: ProMotion Publishing, 1995:43.

Pauling, Linus. *How to Live Longer and Feel Better*. New York: Avon Books, 1986.

Russell RM. "Gastrointestinal function and aging," *Geriatric Nutrition*, JE Morley, ed. New York: Raven Press, 1990:232.

Shils ME, Olson JA, Shike M. *Modern Nutrition in Health and Disease*. 8th ed. Philadelphia: Lea and Febiger, 1994:565.

Suter PM, Russell RM. "Estimate of adequacy of

1989 RDA for vitamins for the elderly. *American Journal of Clinical Nutrition* 45:501–12, 1987.


# Chapter 10: Keeping Your Blood Vessels Strong

Benzer W, et al. "Effects of intravenous magnesium chloride reverses left ventricular end diastolic pressure in coronary artery disease." *American Journal of Cardiology* 77:638–40, 1996 Mar 15.

Bonithon-Knopp C, et al. "Combined effects of lipid peroxidation and antioxidant status on carotid atherosclerosis in a population aged 59–71 years: The EVA study." *American Journal of Clinical Nutrition* 65:121–7, 1997.

Fletcher RH, Fletcher SW. "Glutathione and ageing: ideas and evidence." *Lancet* 344:1379–80, 1994 Nov 19.

Imre SG, MD PhD. "Increased proportion of docosahexanoic acid and high lipid peroxidation capacity in erythrocytes of stroke patients." *Stroke* 25(12):2416–20, 1994.

Knekt P, et al. "Flavonoid intake and coronary mortality in Finland: A cohort study." *British Medical Journal* 312(7029):478–81.

Levine G MD, et al. "Ascorbic acid reverses endothelial vasomotor dysfunction in patients with coronary artery disease." *Circulation* 93(6):1107–13, 1996 Mar 15.

Lip GYH. "Fibrinogen and cardiovascular disorders." *Quarterly Journal of Medicine* 88:155–65, 1995.

McArdle W, Katch F, Katch V. *Exercise Physiology*. Philadelphia/London: Lea and Febiger, 1991.

Muldoon M, Kirtchevsky SB. "Flavonoids and heart disease." *British Medical Journal* 312(7029):458–9, 1996 Feb 24.

O'Keefe J Jr, Lavie C Jr, McCallister B. "Insights into the pathogenesis and prevention of coronary artery disease." *Mayo Clinic Proceedings* 70(1):69–79, 1995 Jan.

Pace-Asciak CR, et al. "Wines and grape juices as modulators of platelet aggregation in healthy human subjects." *Clinica Chimica Acta* 246(1–2):163–82, 1996 Mar 15.

Pauling, Linus. *How to Live Longer and Feel Better*. New York: Avon Books, 1986.

Rath M MD. *Eradicating Heart Disease*. San Francisco: Health Now, 1993.

Stampfer MJ, Malino MR. "Can lowering homocysteine levels reduce cardiovascular risk?" *New England Journal of Medicine* 332(5):328–9, 1995 Feb 2.

Stephens NG, et al. "Randomised controlled study of vitamin E in patients with coronary disease: Cambridge Heart Antioxidant Study(CHAOS)." *Lancet* 347(9004):781–6, 1996 Mar 23.

Torun M, et al. "Serum levels of vitamin E in relation to cardiovascular diseases." *Journal of Clinical Pharmacology* 20:335–40, 1995.

## Chapter 11: Are Your Prescription Drugs Making You Go Blind?

*Drug Facts and Comparisons*. St. Louis: Facts and Comparisons, 1997.

Grahame-Smith DG, Aronson JK. *Oxford Textbook of Clinical Pharmacology and Drug Therapy*. Oxford: Oxford University Press, 1994.

*Physician's Desk Reference*. Montvale, NJ: Medical Economics Data Production Company, 1997.

Wolfe SM MD, Hope R-E RPh. *Worst Pills, Best Pills*. Washington, DC: Public Citizen Health Research Group, 1993.

## Chapter 12: Exercise Your Way to Clear Vision

Barnard R. "Effects of life-style modifications on serum lipids." *Archives of Internal Medicine* 151:1389–94, 1991.

Horton E. "Role and management of exercise in diabetes mellitus." *Diabetes Care* 11:201–11, 1988.

LaPerriere A, et al. "Exercise and psychoneuroim-munology." *Medicine and Science in Sports and Exercise* 26(2):182–90, 1994.

Lee I, Hsieh C, Paffenbarger R. "Exercise intensity and longevity in men: the Harvard Alumni Health Study." *Journal of the American Medical Association* 273:1179–84, 1995.

Lee I, Paffenbarger R. "Physical activity and its relation to cancer risk: A prospective study of college alumni." *Medicine and Science in Sports and Exercise* 26(7):831–37, 1994.

Nash M. "Exercise and immunology." *Medicine and Science in Sports and Exercise* 26(2):125–7, 1994.

Ornish D, et al. "Can lifestyle changes reverse coronary heart disease? The Lifestyle Heart Trial." *Lancet* 336:129–33, 1990.

Pate Russell R, et al. "Physical activity and public health: A recommendation from the Centers for Disease Control and Prevention and the American College of Sports Medicine." *Journal of the American Medical Association* 273(5):402–7, 1995 Feb 1.

Shinkai S, et al. "Physical activity and immune senescence in men." *Medicine and Science in Sports and Exercise* 27(11):1516–26, 1995.

Van Itallie TB MD. "Health implications of overweight and obesity in the United States." *Annals of Internal Medicine* 103(6pt2):983–8, 1985.

# Chapter 13: How to Avoid Vision-Destroying Toxins and Cleanse Your Body of Them

Breen JF, et al. "Coronary artery calcification detected with ultrafast CT as an indication of coronary artery disease." *Radiology* 185(2):435–9, 1992 Nov.

Brillman J. "Central nervous system complications in coronary artery bypass surgery." *Neurologic Clinics* 11(2):475–95, 1993 May.

Cameron AA, Davis KB, Rogers WJ. "Recurrence of angina after coronary artery bypass surgery: Predictors and prognosis (CASS registry), Coronary Artery Surgery Study." *Journal of the American College of Cardiology* 26(4):895–9, 1995 Oct.

Horick P, Smith PL, Taylor KM. "Cerebral complications after coronary bypass grafting." *Current Opinion in Cardiology* 9(6):670–9, 1994 Nov.

Masoro EJ. "Retardation of aging processes by food restriction: An experimental tool." *American Journal of Clinical Nutrition* 55:1250s–2s, 1992.

Nelson JF, et al. "Neuroendocrine involvement in aging: evidence from studies of reproductive aging and caloric restriction." *Neurobiology of Aging* 16(5):837–43; discussion 855–6, 1995 Sep–Oct.

Paul M, Welch L. "Improving education and resources for health care providers." *Environmental Health Perspectives* 101(Suppl2):191–7, 1993 Jul.

Parke DV, Lewis DF. "Safety aspects of food preservatives." *Food Additives and Contaminants* 9(5):561–77, 1992 Sep–Oct.

Pires LA, et al. "Arrhythmias and conduction disturbances after coronary artery bypass graft surgery: epidemiology, management, and prognosis." *American Heart Journal* 129(4):799–808, 1995 Apr.

Wilson JM, Ferguson JJ. "Revascularization therapy for coronary artery disease. Coronary artery bypass grafting versus percutaneous transluminal coronary angioplasty." *Texas Heart Institute Journal* 22(2):145–61, 1995.

## Chapter 14: Basic Eye Care

Baudoin C, et al. "Expression of inflammatory markers by conjunctival cells in chronically treated patients with glaucoma." *Ophthalmology* 101(3):454–60, 1994 Mar.

Gobbels M, Spitznas M. "Corneal epithelial permeability of dry eyes before and after treatment with artificial tears." *Ophthalmology* 99(6):873–8, 1992 Jun.

Jong de C, et al. "Topical timolol with and without benzalkonium chloride." *Graefe's Archives for Clinical and Experimental Ophthalmology* 232(4):221–4, 1994.

Kuppens EV, et al. "Effect of timolol with and without preservative on the basal tear turnover in glaucoma." *British Journal of Ophthalmology* 79(4):339–42, 1995 Apr.

Liu IY, et al. "The association of age-related macular degeneration and lens opacities in the aged." *American Journal of Public Health* 79(6):765–9, 1989 Jun.

Rozanowska M, et al. "Blue light-induced reactivity of retinal age pigment. In vitro generation of oxygen-reactive species." *Journal of Biological Chemistry* 270(32):1822–30, 1995 Aug 11.

# Index

*Page numbers of illustrations appear in italics.*

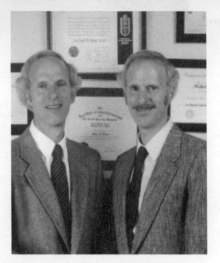

Marc Rose, M.D., and
Michael Rose, M.D.

DR. MARC R. ROSE is a diplomate of the American Board of Ophthalmology and a fellow of the American Academy of Ophthalmology. He did his residency at the University of Illinois Eye and Ear Infirmary, followed by a fellowship for ophthalmic microsurgery at the Texas Medical Center in Houston. He is in private practice specializing in eye health and anti-aging medicine in Los Angeles, West Hollywood, and Costa Mesa, California, with his identical twin, Dr. Michael R. Rose, also an ophthalmologist.

DR. MICHAEL R. ROSE is also a diplomate of the American Board of Ophthalmology and a fellow of the American Academy of Ophthalmology. He did his residency at the Cleveland Clinic in Ohio, followed by a specialty training at Stanford University. He is in private practice specializing in eye health and anti-aging medicine in Los Angeles, West Hollywood, and Costa Mesa, California, with his identical twin, Dr. Marc R. Rose.